Targeting Therapies
in Otitis Media and Otitis Externa

CHARLES D. BLUESTONE, MD

Eberly Professor of Pediatric Otolaryngology
University of Pittsburgh School of Medicine
Director, Department of Pediatric Otolaryngology
Children's Hospital of Pittsburgh
Pittsburgh, PA

MARGARETHA L. CASSELBRANT, MD, PhD

Professor, Department of Otolaryngology
University of Pittsburgh School of Medicine
Director of Research and Education
Department of Pediatric Otolaryngology
Children's Hospital of Pittsburgh
Pittsburgh, PA

JOSEPH E. DOHAR, MD

Associate Professor, Department of Otolaryngology
University of Pittsburgh School of Medicine
Department of Pediatric Otolaryngology
Children's Hospital of Pittsburgh
Pittsburgh, PA

2003
Decker DTC
Hamilton • London

Decker DTC
An Imprint of BC Decker Inc
20 Hughson Street South
P.O. Box 620, LCD 1
Hamilton, Ontario L8N 3K7
Tel: 905-522-7017; 800-568-7281
Fax: 905-522-7839; 888-311-4987
E-mail: info@bcdecker.com
www.bcdecker.com

03 04 05 06/PC/9 8 7 6 5 4 3 2 1

ISBN 1-55009-255-3
Printed in Canada

Sales and Distribution

United States
BC Decker Inc
P.O. Box 785
Lewiston, NY 14092-0785
Tel: 905-522-7017; 800-568-7281
Fax: 905-522-7839; 888-311-4987
E-mail: info@bcdecker.com
www.bcdecker.com

Canada
BC Decker Inc
20 Hughson Street South
P.O. Box 620, LCD 1
Hamilton, Ontario L8N 3K7
Tel: 905-522-7017; 800-568-7281
Fax: 905-522-7839; 888-311-4987
E-mail: info@bcdecker.com
www.bcdecker.com

Foreign Rights
John Scott & Company
International Publishers' Agency
P.O. Box 878
Kimberton, PA 19442
Tel: 610-827-1640
Fax: 610-827-1671
E-mail: jsco@voicenet.com

Japan
Igaku-Shoin Ltd.
Foreign Publications Department
3-24-17 Hongo
Bunkyo-ku, Tokyo, Japan 113-8719
Tel: 3 3817 5680
Fax: 3 3815 6776
E-mail: fd@igaku-shoin.co.jp

*U.K., Europe, Scandinavia,
Middle East*
Elsevier Science
Customer Service Department
Foots Cray High Street
Sidcup, Kent
DA14 5HP, UK
Tel: 44 (0) 208 308 5760
Fax: 44 (0) 181 308 5702
E-mail: cservice@harcourt.com

*Singapore, Malaysia, Thailand,
Philippines, Indonesia, Vietnam,
Pacific Rim, Korea*
Elsevier Science Asia
583 Orchard Road
#09/01, Forum
Singapore 238884
Tel: 65-737-3593
Fax: 65-753-2145

Australia, New Zealand
Elsevier Science Australia
Customer Service Department
STM Division
Locked Bag 16
St. Peters, New South Wales, 2044
Australia
Tel: 61 02 9517-8999
Fax: 61 02 9517-2249
E-mail: stmp@harcourt.com.au
www.harcourt.com.au

Mexico and Central America
ETM SA de CV
Calle de Tula 59
Colonia Condesa
06140 Mexico DF, Mexico
Tel: 52-5-5553-6657
Fax: 52-5-5211-8468
E-mail:editoresdetextosmex@
prodigy.net.mx

Argentina
CLM (Cuspide Libros Medicos)
Av. Córdoba 2067 - (1120)
Buenos Aires, Argentina
Tel: (5411) 4961-0042/
(5411) 4964-0848
Fax: (5411) 4963-7988
E-mail: clm@cuspide.com

Brazil
Tecmedd
Av. Maurílio Biagi, 2850
City Ribeirão Preto – SP – CEP:
14021-000
Tel: 0800 992236
Fax: (16) 3993-9000

DEDICATION

We dedicate this book to our families, teachers, colleagues, house staff, and students, but especially to our patients and their families, whom we hope will benefit from the information contained herein.

ACKNOWLEDGMENT

We wish to acknowledge Maria B. Bluestone for her editorial assistance. We also thank the editors at BC Decker, our publisher, and especially Rochelle Decker, who invited and inspired us to write this unique book.

We are pleased to have collaborated on this text because it is a unique combination of the two most common infections that clinicians encounter: otitis media and otitis externa. To our knowledge, there are no other similar books that combine these two disease entities that are specifically written for clinicians. There are texts dedicated to each of these infections, and both are included in general textbooks of otolaryngology, pediatrics, internal medicine, and infectious diseases. In fact, BC Decker Inc has publications available for each of these infections written by two of us that are specifically for the lay community (Bluestone, 1999, and Dohar, 2002).

It is appropriate to present these two challenging diseases in one text because the clinician is frequently faced with the diagnostic dilemma of deciding if the patient has an infection of the middle ear or the external auditory canal or if both diseases coexist. It is especially difficult for clinicians to make a precise differential diagnosis between the two when otorrhea is the main symptom.

Our knowledge base of both of these entities has advanced significantly during the past few years, especially in management and prevention. These breakthroughs include—but are not limited to—new insights into epidemiology; risk factors; pathogenesis; etiology; new vaccines; and oral, parenteral, and ototopical antimicrobial agents. We also now have ototopical agents that are safe and effective for otorrhea caused by both otitis media and otitis externa.

We have written this text with the primary care physician in mind, but all health care providers who encounter patients with ear disease—otolaryngologists, experts in infectious diseases, allergists, and physician extenders—may benefit from its contents. We hope that the information provided will enhance the health care of patients who have these two common infections.

Charles D. Bluestone, MD
Margaretha L. Casselbrant, MD, PhD
Joseph E. Dohar, MD

ADDITIONAL READINGS

Bluestone CD. Conquering otitis media. Hamilton (ON): BC Decker; 1999.
Dohar JE. Conquering otitis externa. Hamilton (ON): BC Decker; 2002.

CONTENTS

CHAPTER 1

INTRODUCTION

RATIONALE FOR TEXT AND FORMAT

Otitis media and otitis externa are among the most common diagnoses made by primary care physicians. Here we provide the practitioner with methods to distinguish between these two infections.

It is appropriate to combine these two diseases into one text because the clinician is often uncertain which entity is present. This is especially true when the chief complaint is acute or chronic otorrhea. Is the discharge from the ear caused by a perforation in the tympanic membrane (or through a tympanostomy tube) and otitis media, is it caused by an infection in the external auditory canal, or is it caused by both otitis media and otitis externa?

Consider the following:

> When an attack of acute otitis media occurs, a perforation of the tympanic membrane can develop, followed by otorrhea. When a tympanostomy tube is in place, an episode of acute otitis media can also result in otorrhea. These middle ear infections may or may not cause a secondary infection of the ear canal. Chronic otorrhea can also be caused by chronic middle ear (mastoid) infection in which there is a chronic perforation, tympanostomy tube, or a defect such as a retraction pocket or cholesteatoma in the tympanic membrane. As above, this infection may or may not involve the ear canal.
>
> On the other hand, although an episode of acute otitis externa will invariably involve the tympanic membrane, a patient can have a chronic infection of the external ear canal with no middle ear involvement.

Consider also:

> One complication of acute otitis media that can be confused with otitis externa is acute mastoiditis, especially when

there is protrusion of the pinna, postauricular swelling, and erythema. This is because otitis externa may also be present with swelling of the pinna and erythema, tenderness, and swelling of the postauricular area.

The text is divided into three sections. The introductory chapter explains the rationale for combining otitis media and otitis externa into one book, the format of the chapters, and the differential diagnosis of uncomplicated acute otitis media and acute otitis externa. The next section covers otitis media and is followed by a section on otitis externa. In each of these sections (otitis media and otitis externa), we include a chapter on diagnosis.

Even though this text focuses on treatment, other aspects of these diseases, such as epidemiology and pathogenesis, are reviewed to better understand the rationale for treatment and prevention. The last chapter has been devoted to future directions in the various aspects of these diseases and to what is on the horizon for treatment and prevention.

OBJECTIVES

After reading this text, the clinician will

1. Know the current terminology, definitions, and classification of otitis media and otitis externa and the complications and sequelae of otitis media.
2. Learn the current prevalence, incidence, and natural history of, and risk factors for, both diseases.
3. Understand the structure and function of the eustachian tube and how its dysfunction causes otitis media. Be able to explain to parents or caregivers so that they understand how the eustachian tube can be involved in this disease, particularly when it is recurrent or chronic.

4. Learn about the recent advances in our understanding of the pathogenesis of otitis externa, especially related to water exposure during swimming.
5. Learn about the microbiology of otitis media and otitis externa and the current rates of antibiotic-resistant bacterial pathogens related to selecting the most appropriate antimicrobial agents.
6. Clinically distinguish between otitis media and otitis externa.
7. Understand the diagnostic similarities and differences between acute otitis media and otitis media with effusion, which is important in management decisions.
8. Be knowledgeable about the current controversy regarding the question of whether to treat acute otitis media and to realize that severe acute otitis media should be treated with an antimicrobial agent instead of either delaying or withholding such treatment when the disease is mild or most likely to be otitis media with effusion.
9. Select the most appropriate antimicrobial agents for uncomplicated acute otitis media, for example, amoxicillin, leaving the second-line ("backup") drugs for those patients who either have a hypersensitivity to, or are treatment failures with, the currently recommended first-line agent.
10. Learn that persistent, asymptomatic middle ear effusion is common following a course of antimicrobial treatment for acute otitis media and does not require further antibiotic therapy unless the effusion becomes chronic.
11. Be knowledgeable about the timing of the most appropriate medical management options versus "watchful waiting" for the various stages of otitis media with effusion and when referral for consultation with an audiologist and otolaryngologist is appropriate.
12. Determine which ototopical agents are safe and effective for treatment of acute otitis externa, when a wick is

required in the ear canal, and when systemic antimicrobial agents are indicated.

13. Select the safest and most effective ototopical agents for treatment of otorrhea that occurs during an attack of acute otitis media in which the tympanic membrane is not intact.

14. Manage chronic otitis externa with the safest and most effective available treatment.

15. Choose which medical and surgical management options are safest and most effective for prevention of recurrent otitis media and otitis externa and when referral to an otolaryngologist is appropriate.

16. Know the possible complications and sequelae that can occur as a consequence of otitis media and when referral to an otolaryngologist is appropriate.

17. Be aware of what new methods of treatment and prevention of these two common diseases are on the horizon.

SIGNS AND SYMPTOMS ASSOCIATED WITH BOTH OTITIS MEDIA AND OTITIS EXTERNA

The most common signs and symptoms associated with both otitis media and otitis externa may signal another disease or disorder, which can be related or unrelated to otitis. The most common symptom associated with both forms of otitis is *otalgia* and the most common sign associated with both otitis media and otitis externa is *otorrhea*.

Otalgia is pain in the ear, which can be caused by many diseases and disorders, including otitis media and otitis externa (Table 1-1). *Otorrhea* is a discharge from the ear and is frequently encountered in both otic diseases but can be caused by other diseases and disorders (Table 1-2).

The character of the discharge can be helpful in the differential diagnosis between the presence of either otitis media or otitis externa or both versus a source other than the outer and

Table 1–1 Differential Diagnosis of Otalgia

Otologic
  External ear
    Otitis externa
    Impacted cerumen
    Foreign body
    Trauma
    Myringitis
    Perichondritis
    Preauricular cyst/sinus
    Furuncle
    Congenital canal cyst
    Tumor
  Middle ear cleft*
    Acute otitis media
    Otitis media with effusion
    Eustachian tube dysfunction
    Barotrauma
    Mastoiditis
    Tumor

Nonotologic
  Cranial nerves
    III (trigeminal)
      Dental
      Mandible/maxilla
      Temporal mandibular joint
      Oral cavity
      Intratemporal fossa
    VII (facial)
      Bell's palsy
      Herpes zoster oticus (Ramsey Hunt syndrome)
      Tumor
    IX (glossopharyngeal)
      Tonsil
      Hypopharnyx
      Oropharnyx
      Nasopharynx
    X (vagus)
      Hypopharynx
      Larynx
      Esophagus
      Thyroid

Table 1–1 Continued

Gastroesophageal disease
Cervical nerves
Lymph nodes
  Cysts
  Cervical spine
  Neck infections
Other causes
  Neuralgias
  Migraine
  Paranasal sinuses
  Drug induced
  Psychophysiologic
  Munchausen syndrome

Adapted from Dolitsky, 2003.
*Middle ear, eustachian tube, mastoid.

middle ears (Dohar, 2003). Otorrhea that is clear or "watery" can be from the inner ear (perilymphatic fluid) or the intracranial cavity (cerebrospinal fluid), especially if there is copious clear otorrhea following trauma to the ear or head. Although rarely encountered, congenital malformations or tumors of the inner ear or middle ear cleft can also cause the otorrhea. Imaging of the temporal bones and intracranial cavity through computed tomographic scans, radionuclide scanning, or testing the fluid for glucose or β_2-transferrin would provide confirmation. Mucoid, purulent, or mucopurulent drainage usually indicates an infectious etiology. Likewise, bloody or sanguineous drainage usually points to an infectious etiology, but there may be another underlying etiology, such as a tumor.

DIFFERENTIAL DIAGNOSIS BETWEEN OTITIS MEDIA AND OTITIS EXTERNA

At the outset of this book, we provide the reader with the clinical differences between otitis media and otitis externa

Table 1–2   Differential Diagnosis of Otorrhea

External ear
  Otitis externa
  Perichondritis
  Myringitis
  Foreign body
  Herpes zoster oticus (Ramsey Hunt syndrome)
  Congenital canal cyst
  Furuncle
  Trauma
  Cerebrospinal/perilymphatic fluid
  Tumor
  Parotid salivary fluid

Middle ear cleft* (tympanic membrane is nonintact)
  Acute otitis media
  Barotrauma
  Chronic suppurative otitis media
  Cholesteatoma/retraction pocket
  Cerebrospinal/perilymphatic fluid
  Tumor

Inner ear (tympanic membrane is nonintact)
  Cerebrospinal/perilymphatic fluid

*Middle ear, eustachian tube, mastoid.

because the correct diagnosis is essential in providing the safest and most effective treatment.

Acute otitis media is characterized by the rapid onset of signs and symptoms of inflammation within the middle ear, in which one or more local or systemic signs are present: otalgia (or pulling of the ear in the young infant), otorrhea, fever, recent onset of irritability, anorexia, vomiting, or diarrhea. The tympanic membrane is full or bulging, is opaque, and has limited or no mobility to pneumatic otoscopy, all of which indicate middle ear effusion. Erythema of the eardrum is an inconsistent finding. The acute onset of ear pain, fever, and a purulent discharge (otorrhea) through a perforation of the tympanic membrane (or tympanostomy tube) would also be evidence of acute otitis media.

Acute otitis externa is also associated with the rapid onset of the signs and symptoms of inflammation but primarily of the external ear canal and tympanic membrane associated with otalgia and tenderness of the pinna on palpation. Otorrhea is almost always present and is rapidly followed by variable degrees of stenosis of the ear canal. The outer ear may also be involved.

The differential diagnosis between these two disease entities is that when acute otitis media, without otorrhea, is present, the external ear canal is not involved, and there is a lack of tenderness of the pinna. When acute otitis media is the diagnosis, the tympanic membrane has limited or no mobility by pneumatic otoscopy. However, the eardrum is usually mobile (but may have limited mobility) when acute otitis externa is present. Hearing is almost always impaired, to some degree, when otitis media is present owing to the middle ear effusion. When otitis externa is present, hearing loss is not a complaint unless there is moderate to severe canal stenosis. Table 1-3 provides some of the most distinguishing contrasting signs, symptoms, and appearances of the ear.

The problem for the clinician is deciding which disease is present, or when both coexist, when otorrhea is present and the tympanic membrane is difficult to visualize. Is the otorrhea emanating from a perforation of the tympanic membrane or tympanostomy tube, secondary to acute otitis media, or is acute otitis externa the cause of the acute illness? This is particularly difficult when there is any degree of ear canal debris, stenosis, or both and the tympanic membrane is difficult to impossible to visualize. A more complete differential diagnosis is in the chapters devoted to each of these disease entities, in which we also discuss how to obtain an accurate diagnosis or at least a "best guess" when the examination is not optimal. We

	Acute Otitis Media	Acute Otitis Externa
Table 1–3 Acute Otitis Media and Acute Otitis Externa: Most Common Presenting Signs and Symptoms		
Otalgia	Present	Present
Otorrhea	May be present	Usually present
Fever	Usually present	Usually absent
Irritability, anorexia, vomiting, diarrhea	May be present in infants	Uncommon
Tenderness of pinna	Absent	Present
Appearance of TM	Opaque, bulging	Dull, weeping, scaling
Mobility of TM	None or impaired	May be slightly decreased
Dermatitis of meatus, pinna	Absent unless otorrhea	Can be present
Stenosis of ear canal	Absent	Present
Hearing loss	Usually present	Absent without debris/stenosis of ear canal
Tinnitus	May be present	Unusual
Dysequilibrium	May be present	Absent
Cervical lymphadenopathy	Absent	Can be present

TM = tympanic membrane.

also present the differential diagnostic features between the complications of acute otitis media, such as acute mastoiditis, and acute otitis externa in which postauricular cellulitis is present (see Chapter 8, "Complications and Sequelae," in the section on mastoiditis).

When the clinician is uncertain about which disease is involved, especially when the ear canal is very tender and stenotic, or when the tympanic membrane is opaque and a perforation or functioning tympanostomy tube is present, the most prudent management option is to assume that acute otitis media (with otorrhea) and acute otitis externa coexist and treat accordingly. When the patient returns (ideally within a few days) following the treatment, usually with an ototopical agent and a systemic antimicrobial agent, the diagnosis will become more obvious and the systemic antimicrobial agent can be discontinued if the diagnosis is only acute otitis externa (see Chapter 6, "Diagnosis," and Chapter 7, "Management," in this section of the book).

REFERENCES

Bluestone CD. Conquering otitis media. Hamilton (ON): BC Decker; 1999.

Dohar JE. Conquering otitis externa. Hamilton (ON): BC Decker; 2002.

Dohar JE. Otorrhea. In: Bluestone CD, Stool SE, Alper CM, et al, editors. Pediatric otolaryngology. 4th ed. Philadelphia: WB Saunders; 2003. p. 297–305.

Dolitsky JN. Otalgia. In: Bluestone CD, Stool SE, Alper CM, et al, editors. Pediatric otolaryngology, 4th ed. Philadelphia: WB Saunders; 2003. p. 287–95.

CHAPTER 2

TERMINOLOGY, DEFINITIONS, AND CLASSIFICATION

To appropriately target the treatment of otitis media, it is important to learn the currently accepted terminology and definitions of the various types and stages of otitis media and its complications and sequelae. We also provide a classification of these terms related to the clinical presentations and underlying pathology (Bluestone et al, 2002).

TERMINOLOGY AND DEFINITIONS

The terms and definitions that follow are the ones most commonly used in relation to otitis media:

Otitis media is an inflammation of the middle ear cleft without reference to etiology or pathogenesis.

Acute otitis media is the rapid onset of signs and symptoms, such as otalgia and fever, of acute infection within the middle ear.

Otitis media with effusion is an inflammation of the middle ear with a collection of liquid in the middle ear space. The signs and symptoms of acute infection are absent, and there is no perforation of the tympanic membrane or otorrhea.

Middle ear effusion designates a liquid in the middle ear but not etiology, pathogenesis, pathology, or duration. An effusion may be serous, a thin, watery liquid; mucoid, a thick, viscid, mucus-like liquid; purulent, a pus-like liquid; or a combination of these. An effusion can be the result of either acute otitis media or otitis media with effusion. The effusion can be of recent onset, acute, or more long-lasting, subacute, or chronic.

Persistent middle ear effusion is an effusion that persists in the middle ear following an episode of acute otitis media.

Otorrhea is a discharge from the ear originating at one or more of the following sites: external auditory canal, middle ear, mastoid, inner ear, or intracranial cavity.

Recurrent acute otitis media is defined as three or more episodes in the previous 6 months or four or more in the past 12 months, with one in the recent past.

The following are definitions of the intratemporal (extracranial) complications and sequelae of otitis media, which are those that occur within the temporal bone.

Hearing loss can be either partial or complete, transient or permanent, and conductive, sensorineural, or both.

Vertigo is defined as a subjective sensation of movement of the patient or the surroundings, such as spinning, turning, or whirling. Vertigo can be either acute, recurrent, or chronic.

Dizziness is a nonspecific term describing a sensation of altered orientation to the environment, which may or may not be true vertigo.

Perforation of the tympanic membrane is a nonintact tympanic membrane, which can be either acute or chronic.

Chronic suppurative otitis media is chronic infection of the middle ear and mastoid air cells in which there is a nonintact tympanic membrane and otorrhea.

Mastoiditis is an inflammation of the mastoid air cell system and can be either acute, subacute, or chronic.

Petrositis is an inflammation in the mastoid apex cells. It is also called *petrous apicitis* or *apical petrositis*.

Labyrinthitis is an inflammation in the cochlear and vestibular apparatus and can be acute or chronic and transient or permanent.

Facial paralysis is a paralysis of the facial muscles and can be acute or chronic, partial or complete, and transient or permanent.

Otitis externa is an infection of the external auditory canal and can be a complication of otitis media (with perforation or tympanostomy tube and otorrhea). It can also be present in the absence of otitis media.

Atelectasis of the middle ear is retraction or collapse of the tympanic membrane and may be acute or chronic, localized (with or without a *retraction pocket*) or generalized, and mild, moderate, or severe.

Adhesive otitis media occurs when the mucous membrane within the middle ear is thickened by proliferation of fibrous tissue. This frequently impairs movement of the ossicles, resulting in conductive hearing loss.

Cholesteatoma is a keratinizing, stratified squamous epithelium that accumulates in the middle ear or other pneumatized portions of the temporal bone. The term *aural* distinguishes this type of cholesteatoma from a similar pathologic entity that occurs outside the temporal bone. *Acquired* distinguishes it as a sequela of otitis media or related conditions (eg, retraction pocket of the tympanic membrane) distinct from aural congenital cholesteatomas. Even though this term is a misnomer—*keratoma* is more consistent with the pathology—cholesteatoma is in common use.

Cholesterol granuloma is tissue composed of chronic granulations with foreign body giant cells, foam cells, and cholesterol crystals within the middle ear, mastoid, or both.

Tympanosclerosis is whitish plaques in the tympanic membrane (ie, myringosclerosis) and nodular deposits in the submucosal layers of the middle ear.

Ossicular discontinuity is rarefying osteitis resulting in disarticulation of one or both ossicular joints or any portion of the ossicles causing disarticulation.

Ossicular fixation is caused by fibrous tissue from adhesive otitis media, tympanosclerosis, or both. The ossicle itself or one of the joints (ie, incudostapedial or incudomalleolar) may be fixed.

The following are the intracranial suppurative complications of otitis media. These may be caused by one or more of the intratemporal complications, such as labyrinthitis or mastoiditis, or one or more of the other complications of otitis media within the intracranial cavity.

Otitic meningitis is an inflammation of the meninges that, when it is a suppurative complication of otitis media or certain related conditions (eg, labyrinthitis), is usually caused by a bacterium associated with infections of the middle ear, mastoid, or both.

Extradural abscess, also called *epidural abscess*, is an infection that occurs between the dura of the brain and the cranial bone.

Subdural empyema is a collection of purulent material within the potential space between the dura externally and the arachnoid membrane internally. Because the pus collects in a preformed space, it is correctly termed *empyema* rather than *abscess*.

Focal otitic encephalitis (also called *cerebritis*) is a focal area of the brain that is edematous and inflamed. The signs and symptoms of this complication are similar to those associated with a brain abscess.

Otogenic brain abscess is a suppuration within the brain as a complication of otitis media–mastoiditis or one or more of its other complications, such as otitic meningitis.

Lateral and *sigmoid sinus thrombosis* or *thrombophlebitis* is inflammation with thrombus formation within dural sinuses as a result of otitis media, an intratemporal complication such as acute mastoiditis or apical petrositis, or another intracranial complication of otitis media.

Otitic hydrocephalus is a complication of otitis media in which there is increased intracranial pressure without abnormalities of cerebrospinal fluid. The term *benign intracranial hypertension* also seems appropriate.

CLASSIFICATION

A classification of otitis media and its complications and sequelae are listed in Table 2-1. Initially, otitis media is classified into *acute otitis media* and *otitis media with effusion* and its related disorder, *eustachian tube dysfunction*. Complications and sequelae of otitis media are classified into *intratemporal* (extracranial) complications and sequelae, which are those that occur within the

Table 2–1   Classification of Otitis Media
Initial Presentation
Acute otitis media
Otitis media with effusion
Acute (short duration)
Subacute
Chronic
Eustachian tube dysfunction
Intratemporal (Extracranial) Complications and Sequelae
Hearing loss (conductive, sensorineural, or both)
Vestibular, balance, and motor dysfunctions

Table 2–1   Continued

Perforation of tympanic membrane
  Acute perforation without or without otorrhea
  Chronic perforation with acute otitis media (with or without otorrhea)
  Chronic suppurative otitis media
Mastoiditis
  Acute
    Acute mastoiditis without periosteitis/osteitis
    Acute mastoiditis with periosteitis
    Acute mastoiditis with osteitis
      Without subperiosteal abscess
      With subperiosteal abscess
  Subacute
  Chronic
Apical petrositis
Labyrinthitis
  Acute
  Chronic
  Labyrinthine ossificans
Facial paralysis
  Acute
  Chronic
External otitis
  Acute
  Chronic
Atelectasis of the middle ear
  With or without retraction pocket
Adhesive otitis media
Cholesteatoma
Cholesterol granuloma
Tympanosclerosis
Ossicular discontinuity
Ossicular fixation

Intracranial Complications
  Meningitis
  Extradural abscess
  Subdural empyema
  Focal otitic encephalitis
  Brain abscess
  Dural sinus thrombosis
  Otitic hydrocephalus

temporal bone, and *intracranial*, which are those that occur within the intracranial cavity. The clinical descriptions and signs and symptoms of each of these entities are described in detail in Chapter 6, "Diagnosis," and Chapter 8, "Complications and Sequelae."

REFERENCE

Bluestone CD, Gates GA, Klein JO, et al. Chairman: committee report: terminology and classification of otitis media and its complications and sequelae. In: Lim DJ, Bluestone CD, Casselbrant ML, et al, editors. Seventh International Symposium on Recent Advances in Otitis Media: report of the research conference. Ann Otol Rhinol Laryngol 2002;111(3 Suppl 188, Pt 2):8–18.

CHAPTER 3

EPIDEMIOLOGY

To target management of otitis media, it is appropriate to have an understanding of the risk factors associated with the disease, especially when the patient has recurrent acute otitis media, recurrent/chronic middle ear effusion, or both. Table 3-1 lists these risk factors.

HOST-RELATED FACTORS

Age

The highest incidence of acute otitis media occurs between 6 and 11 months of age (Teele et al, 1989). Onset of the first episode of acute otitis media before 6 months of age is a powerful predictor of recurrent acute otitis media.

The risk for persistent middle ear effusion after an episode of acute otitis media is also inversely correlated with age. Shurin and colleagues (1979) found the risk for persistent middle ear effusion after acute otitis media to be four times higher in children under 2 years of age than in older children. Marchisio and colleagues (1988) followed 196 Italian children for 3 months after an episode of acute otitis media and found that younger children were significantly more likely to develop chronic middle ear effusion than were older children.

Children experiencing their first episode of middle ear effusion before 2 months of age were found to be at higher risk for persistent effusion (3 months or longer) during their first year of life than were children who had their first episode later.

Prematurity

Some studies have found an increased risk of middle ear effusion in premature infants, whereas others have not. Gravel

Table 3–1 Risk Factors Associated with Recurrent Acute Otitis Media and Recurrent/Chronic Middle Ear Effusions

Host Related
  Age
  Prematurity
  Gender
  Race
  Allergy
  Immunocompetence
  Craniofacial abnormalities
  Genetic predisposition

Environmental
  Upper respiratory tract infections
  Season
  Day care
  Siblings
  Passive smoking
  Breast-feeding
  Socioeconomic status
  Pacifier use

and colleagues (1988), in a prospective study of 49 children who had been in the newborn intensive care unit and 19 full-term infants, did not find any association between gestational age, birth weight, or length of stay in the intensive care unit and percentage of visits with middle ear effusion during the first year of life. Alho and colleagues (1990) examined the records of 2,512 children from birth to 2 years of age and found no association between acute otitis media and low birth weight (< 2,500 g) or prematurity (< 37 weeks). Engel and colleagues (1999), in a prospective study of 150 full-term and 100 high-risk infants (most preterm or very low birth weight infants), found higher prevalence rates of otitis media with effusion in the high-risk group. Peak prevalence was 59% in the high-risk group versus 49% in the full-term group, which was observed around the age of 10 months in both groups.

Gender

Most investigators have reported no apparent gender-based difference in the incidence of otitis media with effusion or in time with middle ear effusion (Paradise et al, 1997). Some studies have found males to have a significantly higher incidence of acute otitis media and more recurrent episodes of acute otitis media than females (Teele et al, 1989), but others have not found males to have more episodes of acute otitis media (Casselbrant et al, 1995). Males have been reported to be more prone to persistent middle ear effusion. The reason for the sex difference is not known.

Race

Previous studies have suggested a lower incidence of otitis media in African American children compared with American white children (Schappert, 1992; Shurin et al, 1979). In a report from the Division of Health Care Statistics (Schappert, 1992), the office visit rate for otitis media was much lower for black children compared with that for white children. However, in a recent prospective study, no difference was found between black children and white children in their experience with otitis media when the children were from the same socioeconomic background, were examined at monthly intervals and whenever they developed signs and symptoms of ear disease, and received the same treatment for ear disease from birth to 2 years of age (Casselbrant et al, 1995). In another prospective study, 2,253 children were followed from approximately 2 months to 2 years of age, with otoscopic examinations every 6 weeks. The mean cumulative percentage of days with middle ear effusion during the first year was higher in the black infants than in the white infants, but by the second year, the rates were equal (Paradise et al, 1997).

Also, there are certain racial groups in the world that have a higher incidence of otitis media than others. The Aborigines of Australia and some Native Americans (Inuit, Apache, and Navajo) have a higher incidence than the white population. Their underlying susceptibility may be either immunologic or eustachian tube dysfunction or some other unrecognized factors (Bluestone, 1998).

Allergy and Immunity

Allergy is a common problem in young children, occurring at a time when respiratory viral infections and otitis media are both very prevalent. There is still controversy regarding the role of allergy in the pathogenesis of otitis media. Several mechanisms have been suggested, including the middle ear functioning as a "shock organ," inflammatory swelling of the eustachian tube, and inflammatory obstruction of the nose and secondary eustachian tube dysfunction (Bluestone, 1983).

Evidence that allergic rhinitis contributes to the pathogenesis of middle ear effusion is derived from epidemiologic, mechanistic, and therapeutic lines of investigation. Kraemer and colleagues (1983) compared risk factors for persistent middle ear effusion among 76 children admitted for bilateral myringotomy and tube insertion and 76 controls matched by age, sex, and season of admission for a general surgical procedure. They showed a nearly fourfold increase in the risk of persistent middle ear effusion in children who had atopic symptoms for more than 15 days per month. Pukander and Karma (1988) followed 707 children with acute otitis media and found persistence of middle ear effusion for 2 months or more to be greater in children with "atopic manifestations" (undefined) than in children without allergy. In another study, however, allergic manifestations were not found to predispose a child to develop acute otitis media.

Human immunodeficiency virus (HIV)-infected children have a significantly higher recurrence rate of acute otitis media than normal children (Principi et al, 1991) or children who seroconverted (Barnett et al, 1992). Infected children with a low CD4 lymphocyte count had a nearly threefold increased risk for recurrent acute otitis media compared with HIV-infected children with normal lymphocyte counts.

Cleft Palate, Craniofacial Abnormality, Down Syndrome, and Eustachian Tube Dysfunction

Otitis media is present in nearly all infants under 2 years of age with unrepaired clefts of the palate (Paradise and Bluestone, 1974). The occurrence of otitis media was reduced following surgical repair of the palate (Paradise and Bluestone, 1974), likely owing to improvement of the eustachian tube function (Doyle et al, 1986). Otitis media is also common in children with craniofacial abnormalities and Down syndrome (Balkany et al, 1978). The children with Down syndrome have, in addition to poor active opening function of the eustachian tube, a very low resistance of the tube. Secretions from the nasopharynx can therefore easily access the middle ear (White et al, 1984). But individuals who have recurrent acute/chronic middle ear disease and who do not have a craniofacial malformation also can have dysfunction of the eustachian tube, which is described in detail in Chapter 4, "Pathogenesis."

Genetic

The frequency of one episode of otitis media occurring is so high that a genetic predisposition cannot be expected. However, a predisposition to recurrent episodes of otitis media and chronic middle ear effusion may have a significant genetic component. Anatomic, physiologic, and epidemiologic data suggest this. For example, the degree of pneumatization of the mastoid process, a trait believed to be linked causally to otitis media, was found to be more similar in monozygotic than dizygotic twins (Dahlberg and Diamant, 1945). Racial differences in eustachian tube anatomy and function have also been reported. The shorter, straighter eustachian tube found in American Indians is associated with a higher incidence of chronic suppurative otitis media (Doyle, 1977). In a study of Apache Indians adopted into middle-class foster homes, Spivey and Hirschhorn (1977) found that the incidence of most infectious diseases decreased, but the incidence of otitis media was comparable to that reported for the reservation.

Familial clustering of otitis media suggests a genetic component to the disease (Stenström and Ingvarsson, 1997). Rich and colleagues (1994), using tympanostomy tube placement as the basis for proband identification, estimated that the genetic component accounted for up to 60% of otitis media liability in a "permissive environment."

Twin and triplet studies have been used to assess heritability for otitis media. Two retrospective questionnaire studies have been reported. The first study of 2,750 Norwegian twin pairs estimated the heritability at 74% in females and 45% in males (Kvaerner et al, 1997). In the second study, the estimated heritability at ages 2, 3, and 4 years for acute infections was, on average, 57% (Rovers et al, 2002). In a prospective twin/triplet study from Pittsburgh, with monthly assessment of middle ear status, the heritability estimate for otitis media at age 2 years was 79% in females and 64% in males (Casselbrant et al, 1999).

ENVIRONMENTAL FACTORS

Season and Upper Respiratory Infection

Both epidemiologic evidence and clinical experience strongly suggest that otitis media is frequently a complication of upper respiratory infection. The incidence of otitis media with effusion is highest during the fall and winter months and lowest in the summer months in both the northern and southern hemispheres, which parallels the incidence of acute otitis media and upper respiratory infection (Casselbrant et al, 1985). This supports the hypothesis that an episode of upper respiratory infection plays an important role in the etiology of otitis media. Experimental (Buchman et al, 1994) and clinical (Bylander, 1984) studies have shown that viral upper respiratory infection is a risk factor for eustachian tube dysfunction and development of otitis media.

Upper respiratory tract infections with respiratory syncytial virus, influenza virus, and adenovirus often precede episodes of acute otitis media. Respiratory syncytial virus, rhinovirus, adenovirus, and coronavirus have been isolated in episodes of acute otitis media.

Day Care/Home Care

Almost universally, studies identify daycare center attendance as a very important risk factor for developing otitis media, possibly explained by the increased risk for upper respiratory infection in young children in day care (Wald et al, 1988). Children in daycare centers are at increased risk for upper respiratory infection probably because of the large number of susceptible children in close contact.

Prevalence of high negative middle ear pressure and flat tympanograms (type B), indicative of middle ear effusion, has been shown to be highest in children cared for in daycare centers with many children, intermediate in children in family day care with fewer children, and lowest in children cared for at home. Children cared for in a daycare center for at least 12 months during the first 4 years of life have 2.6 times the risk of developing persistent otitis media with effusion compared with children cared for at home.

Alho and colleagues (1993) examined responses to questionnaires sent to parents of 2,512 Finnish children as well as the children's medical records and found an odds ratio of 2.06 for the development of acute otitis media in children attending daycare centers compared with children cared for at home. This increased incidence of acute otitis media in children in daycare centers was also found in a case-control study in Finland (Pukander and Karma, 1988). Children in day care have also been shown to be more likely to have a tympanostomy tube inserted than children cared for at home (Wald et al, 1988).

Siblings

Birth order was associated with the rate of episodes of otitis media and percentage of time with middle ear effusion in a prospective longitudinal study by Casselbrant and colleagues (1995). The study found that firstborn children had a lower rate of acute otitis media and less time with middle ear effusion during the first 2 years of life than did children with older siblings. Pukander and colleagues (1988) also found that children with more siblings were most likely to have recurrent episodes of acute otitis media. Having more than one sibling was significantly related to early onset of otitis media. However, Teele and colleagues (1989) reported no association between the number of siblings and the risk for acute otitis media or middle ear effusion.

The reason for the higher morbidity is probably the same as for children in day care. Paradise and colleagues (1997) combined the number of older siblings and daycare attendance into a "child exposure index" and found a significant correlation with cumulative time with middle ear effusion. The more children in the same place, the greater the opportunity for exposure to upper respiratory infection, which may cause eustachian tube dysfunction and increase the likelihood of developing otitis media.

Passive Smoking

An association between otitis media and passive exposure to smoking has been reported by many investigators (Etzel et al, 1992). The risk of recurrent otitis media (more than six lifetime episodes) was significantly increased with combined gestational and passive smoke exposure.

In most studies, information on smoke exposure has been obtained from the parents' report. Strachan and colleagues (1989), however, measured cotinine, a metabolite of nicotine and a marker of passive exposure to smoking, in the saliva of children 6 to 7 years of age and correlated its concentration with middle ear status as determined by tympanometry. They found that increased cotinine concentrations correlated with abnormal tympanograms and the number of smokers in the household.

Etzel and colleagues (1992) measured serum cotinine concentration in children who attended a daycare center. Children exposed to tobacco smoke who had a serum cotinine concentration > 2.5 ng/mL had a 38% higher rate of new episodes of middle ear effusion and otitis media episodes of longer duration.

Breast-feeding versus Bottle Feeding

Most studies have found that breast-feeding has a protective effect against middle ear disease. However, there is controversy regarding the duration of breast-feeding necessary for protection. Some investigators have found no association between duration of breast-feeding and recurrence rate of acute otitis media, but many have reported fewer recurrences of acute otitis media among children who were breast-fed exclusively for a prolonged period of time. Duncan and colleagues (1993) followed 1,013 infants in a 1-year study and found that infants exclusively breast-fed for 4 months or longer had half the mean number of acute otitis media episodes compared with infants who were not breast-fed at all and 40% less than infants breast-fed less than 4 months. The recurrence rate in infants exclusively breast-fed for 6 months or longer was 10% compared with 20.5% in infants who were breast-fed less than 4 months.

The mechanism for the protective effect of breast milk is not known, but several hypotheses have been suggested. The protective mechanism may be through immunologic factors provided through the breast milk, especially secretory immunoglobulin A, with antibody activity against respiratory tract viruses and bacteria, or it may be through other factors preventing bacterial adhesion (Andersson et al, 1986). Bluestone and Klein (2001) have suggested mechanisms in bottle-fed children that may account for these differences, including allergy to formula or cow's milk, poorer development of facial musculature needed to promote good eustachian tube function, aspiration of fluids in the middle ear with high intraoral pressures generated by bottle feeding, and the reclining or horizontal position of the infants during feeding possibly causing reflux.

Socioeconomic Status

Socioeconomic status and access to health care are factors that may affect the incidence of otitis media. It has generally been thought that otitis media is more common among people in the lower socioeconomic strata owing to poor sanitary conditions and crowding. Paradise and colleagues (1997) followed 2,253 infants for 2 years and found an inverse relationship between the cumulative proportion of days with middle ear effusion and socioeconomic status. However, many studies revealed no correlation between socioeconomic status of the child's family and incidence of middle ear effusion.

Pacifier Use

Niemelä and colleagues (1994) found from parental questionnaires that among 938 5-year-old children, those who had
used a pacifier had a greater risk of having had four or more
episodes of acute otitis media than those who had not,
whereas thumb sucking was not associated with acute otitis
media. In a follow-up prospective study of 845 children in
daycare centers, Niemelä and colleagues (1995) found that use
of a pacifier increased the annual incidence of acute otitis
media and calculated that pacifier use was responsible for 25%
of acute otitis media episodes in children younger than 3 years.

CONCLUSION

We conclude that there are evidence-based risk factors that
are associated with recurrent acute otitis media and chronic/
recurrent middle ear effusion and that the clinician should
inform the parents/caretakers regarding the factors that can be
instituted to reduce the rate for each. These include a search
for an underlying allergy, immunologic immaturity, or disorder
or placing an infant or young child in a daycare setting with
the fewest number of children as possible. It might also include
eliminating day care, smoking in the household, and pacifier
use past the age of 1 year. Even though a child who is not
breast-fed and has recurrent or chronic disease cannot be
changed to breast-feeding, the mother can be informed about
the genetic aspects of otitis media and encouraged to breast-
feed any future children. Also, parents/caretakers can be
informed about factors that they have relatively no control
over—prematurity, male gender, eustachian tube dysfunction,
craniofacial abnormalities, genetic predisposition, youngest
sibling—to better understand their child's recurrent/chronic
middle ear infections.

REFERENCES

Álho O, Kilkku O, Oja H, et al. Control of the temporal aspect when considering risk factors for acute otitis media. Arch Otolaryngol Head Neck Surg 1993;119:444–9.

Alho O, Koivu M, Hartikainen-Sorri A, et al. Is a child's history of acute otitis media and respiratory infection already determined in the antenatal and perinatal period? Int J Pediatr Otorhinolaryngol 1990;19:129–37.

Andersson B, Porras O, Hanson LA, et al. Inhibition of attachment of *Streptococcus pneumoniae* and *Haemophilus influenzae* by human milk and receptor oligosaccharides. J Infect Dis 1986;153:232–7.

Balkany TJ, Downs MP, Jafek BW, Krajicek MJ. Otologic manifestations of Down syndrome. Surg Forum 1978;29:582–5.

Barnett ED, Klein JO, Pelton SI, Luginbuhl LM. Otitis media in children born to human immunodeficiency virus-infected mothers. Pediatr Infect Dis J 1992;11:360–4.

Bluestone CD. Epidemiology and pathogenesis of chronic suppurative otitis media: implications for prevention and treatment. Int J Pediatr Otorhinolaryngol 1998;42:207–23.

Bluestone CD. Eustachian tube function: physiology, pathophysiology, and role of allergy in pathogenesis of otitis media. J Allergy Clin Immunol 1983;72:242–51.

Bluestone CD, Klein JO. Otitis media in infants and children. 3rd ed. Philadelphia: WB Saunders; 2001. p. 49–51.

Buchman CA, Doyle WJ, Skoner D, et al. Otologic manifestations of experimental rhinovirus infection. Laryngoscope 1994;104: 1295–9.

Bylander A. Upper respiratory tract infection and eustachian tube function in children. Acta Otolaryngol (Stockh) 1984;97:343–9.

Casselbrant ML, Brostoff LM, Cantekin EI, et al. Otitis media with effusion in preschool children. Laryngoscope 1985;95:428–36.

Casselbrant ML, Mandel EM, Fall PA, et al. The heritability of otitis media: a twin and triplet study. JAMA 1999;282:2125–30.

Casselbrant ML, Mandel EM, Kurs-Lasky M, et al. Otitis media in a population of black American and white American infants, 0–2 years of age. Int J Pediatr Otorhinolaryngol 1995;33:1–16.

Dahlberg G, Diamant M. Hereditary character in the cellular system of the mastoid process. Acta Otolaryngol (Stockh) 1945;33:378–89.

Doyle WJ. A functional-anatomic description of eustachian tube vector relations in four ethnic populations: an osteologic study [PhD dissertation]. Pittsburgh: University of Pittsburgh; 1977.

Doyle WJ, Reilly JS, Jardini L, Rovnak S. Effect of palatoplasty on the function of the eustachian tube in children with cleft palate. Cleft Palate J 1986;23:63–8.

Duncan B, Ey J, Holberg CJ, et al. Exclusive breastfeeding for at least 4 months protects against otitis media. Pediatrics 1993;91:867–72.

Engel J, Anteunis L, Volovics A, et al. Prevalence rates of otitis media with effusion from 0 to 2 years of age: healthy-born versus high-risk-born infants. Int J Pediatr Otorhinolaryngol 1999;47:243–51.

Etzel RA, Pattishall EN, Haley NJ, et al. Passive smoking and middle-ear effusion among children in day care. Pediatrics 1992;90: 228–32.

Gravel JS, McCarton CM, Ruben RJ. Otitis media in neonatal intensive care unit graduates: a 1-year prospective study. Pediatrics 1988;82: 44–9.

Kraemer MJ, Richardson MA, Weiss NS, et al. Risk factors for persistent middle-ear effusions—otitis media, catarrh, cigarette smoke exposure, and atopy. JAMA 1983;249:1022–5.

Kvaerner KJ, Harris JR, Tambs K, Magnus P. Distribution and heritability of recurrent ear infections. Ann Otol Rhinol Laryngol 1997; 106:624–32.

Marchisio P, Bigalli L, Massironi E, Principi N. Risk factors for persisting otitis media with effusion in children. In: Lim DJ, Bluestone CD, Klein JO, Nelson JD, editors. Recent advances in otitis media with effusion. Proceedings of the Fourth International Symposium. Philadelphia: BC Decker; 1988. p. 3–5.

Niemelä M, Uhari M, Hannuksela A. Pacifiers and dental structure as risk factors for otitis media. Int J Pediatr Otorhinolaryngol 1994; 29:121–7.

Niemelä M, Uhari M, Möttönen M. A pacifier increases the risk of recurrent acute otitis media in children in day-care centers. Pediatrics 1995;96:884–8.

Paradise JL, Bluestone CD. Early treatment of the universal otitis media of infants with cleft palate. Pediatrics 1974;53:48–54.

Paradise JL, Rockette HE, Colburn K, et al. Otitis media in 2253 Pittsburgh-area infants: prevalence and risk factors during the first two years of life. Pediatrics 1997;99:318–33.

Principi N, Marchisio P, Tornaghi R, et al. Acute otitis media in human immunodeficiency virus-infected children. Pediatrics 1991;88: 566–71.

Pukander JS, Karma PH. Persistence of middle-ear effusion and its risk factors after an acute attack of otitis media with effusion. In: Lim DJ, Bluestone CD, Klein JO, Nelson JD, editors. Recent advances in otitis media. Proceedings of the Fourth International Symposium. Philadelphia: BC Decker; 1988. p. 8–11.

Rich SS, Savona K, Giebink GS, Daly K. Familial aggregation and risk factors for chronic/recurrent otitis media. Am J Hum Genet 1994; 55:942.

Rovers M, Haggard M, Gannon M, et al. Heritability of symptom domains in otitis media: a longitudinal study of 1,373 twin pairs. Am J Epidemiol 2002;155:958–64.

Schappert SM. Office visits for otitis media: United States, 1975–90. Adv Data 1992;214:1–19.

Shurin PA, Pelton SI, Donner A, Klein JO. Persistence of middle-ear effusion after acute otitis media in children. N Engl J Med 1979; 300:1121–3.

Spivey GH, Hirschhorn N. A migrant study of adopted Apache children. Johns Hopkins Med J 1977;1210:43–6.

Stenström C, Ingvarsson L. Otitis-prone children and controls: a study of possible predisposing factors. I. Heredity, family background and perinatal period. Acta Otolaryngol (Stockh) 1997;117:87–93.

Strachan DP, Jarvis MJ, Feyerabend C. Passive smoking, salivary cotinine concentrations, and middle ear effusion in 7 year old children. BMJ 1989;298:1549–52.

Teele DW, Klein JO, Rosner B, Greater Boston Otitis Media Study Group. Epidemiology of otitis media during the first seven years of life in children in greater Boston: a prospective, cohort study. J Infect Dis 1989;160:83–94.

Wald ER, Dashefsky B, Byers C, et al. Frequency and severity of infections in day care. J Pediatr 1988;112:540–6.

White BL, Doyle WJ, Bluestone CD. Eustachian tube function in infants and children with Down syndrome. In: Lim DJ, Bluestone CD, Klein JO, Nelson JD, editors. Recent advances in otitis media with effusion. Proceedings of the Third International Symposium. Philadelphia: BC Decker; 1984. p. 62–6.

CHAPTER 4

PATHOGENESIS

An understanding of the normal and abnormal function of the eustachian tube can help the clinician target the treatment of otitis media, especially when the disease becomes chronic and recurrent. The pathogenesis of otitis media is multifactorial, which includes one or more of the following: eustachian tube dysfunction and genetic, infectious, immunologic, allergic, environmental, and social factors (Figure 4-1).

The most important factors related to the increased incidence of otitis media in infants and young children are a functionally and structurally immature eustachian tube and an immature immune system. A genetic predisposition is also critical in many infants and children (Casselbrant et al, 1999). The following is a review of the normal and abnormal function of the eustachian tube within its middle ear system, which includes the nasopharynx, the nasal cavities at its anterior end, and the middle ear and mastoid cells at its posterior end (Figure 4-2).

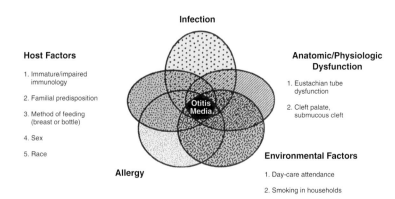

Figure 4–1 Factors involved in the etiology and pathogenesis of otitis media. Reproduced with permission from Bluestone CD, Stool SE, Alper CM, et al, editors. Pediatric otolaryngology. 4th ed. Philadelphia: WB Saunders; 2003.

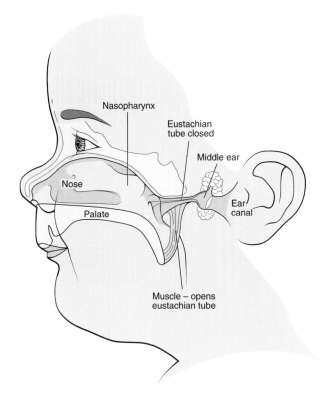

Figure 4–2 The eustachian tube–middle-ear system in which the pharynx, palate, and nasal cavities are proximal to the tube and, at the distal end, the middle ear and mastoid cells. Reproduced with permission from Bluestone CD. Conquering otitis media. Hamilton (ON): BC Decker; 1999.

NORMAL FUNCTION

There are three physiologic functions attributed to the eustachian tube: (1) *pressure regulation* (ventilation) of the middle ear that equilibrates gas pressure in the middle ear with atmospheric pressure, (2) *protection* of the middle ear from nasopharyngeal sound pressure and secretions, and (3) *clearance* (drainage) of secretions produced within the middle ear into the nasopharynx. The tube actively opens during swallowing owing to the contraction of the tensor veli palatini muscle.

The most important of the three functions of the eustachian tube is regulation of pressure (ventilation) within the middle ear. This is because hearing is optimal when middle ear gas pressure is relatively the same as air pressure in the external auditory canal, that is, tympanic membrane and middle ear mobility is optimal. The tube actively opens during swallowing owing to the contraction of the tensor veli palatini muscle (Figure 4-3).

The protective function prevents unwanted secretions from the nasopharynx from gaining entrance into the middle

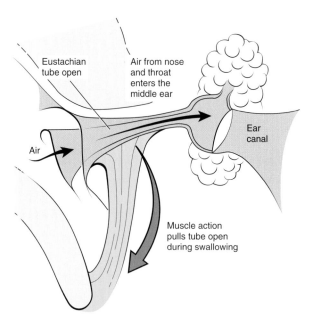

Figure 4–3 Pressure regulation function. During swallowing, the eustachian tube opens by the contraction of the tensor veli palatini muscle, which equilibrates pressure between the outside atmosphere (nasopharynx) and the middle ear. Reproduced from Bluestone CD. Conquering otitis media. Hamilton (ON): BC Decker; 1999.

ear, which may cause middle ear infection and can decrease hearing. The eustachian tube system helps protect the middle ear and mastoid cell system through its functional anatomy and through the immunologic and mucociliary defense of its mucous membrane lining. Protection of the middle ear from abnormal nasopharyngeal sound pressures and secretions depends on the normal structure and function of the eustachian tube and the ability of the middle ear and mastoid cell system to maintain a "*gas cushion.*" Tubal anatomy, in which the narrow portion (isthmus) of the tube is in the middle, and the middle ear gas cushion inhibit reflux of secretions from the nasopharynx into the middle ear (Figure 4-4).

Clearance (drainage) of secretions from the middle ear into the nasopharynx is provided by two physiologic methods: mucociliary clearance and muscular clearance. The mucocil-

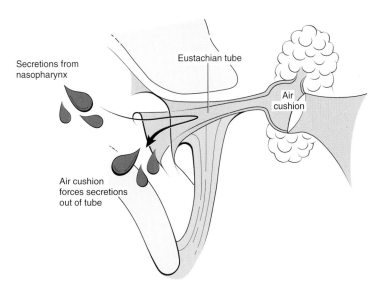

Figure 4–4 Protective function of the eustachian tube. Reproduced from Bluestone CD. Conquering otitis media. Hamilton (ON): BC Decker; 1999.

iary system of the eustachian tube and some areas of the middle ear mucous membrane clear secretions from the middle ear, and the *"pumping action"* of the eustachian tube during closing provides the other method. Other factors, such as surface tension–lowering substances, similar to the lung, may contribute to optimal normal opening of the eustachian tube (Figure 4-5).

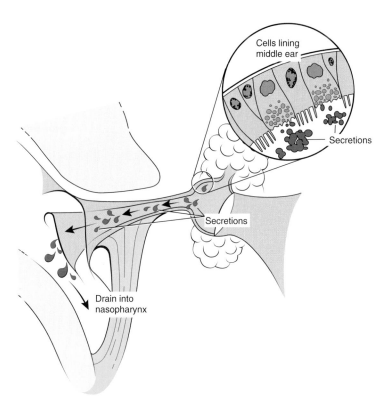

Figure 4–5 Clearance (drainage) function. The eustachian tube pumps out secretions from the tube and the middle ear into the nasopharynx. Also, the mucociliary system in the tube and the middle ear aids in clearance. Reproduced from Bluestone CD. Conquering otitis media. Hamilton (ON): BC Decker; 1999.

ABNORMAL FUNCTION

As depicted in Figure 4-6, abnormal function of the eustachian tube system can be simply described as follows (Bluestone, 1999):

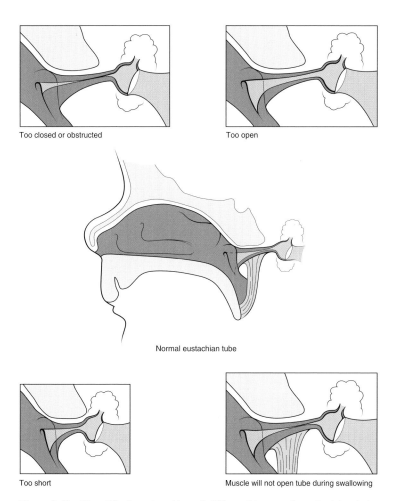

Figure 4–6 Simplified explanation of different types of eustachian tube dysfunction. Reproduced from Bluestone CD. Conquering otitis media. Hamilton (ON): BC Decker; 1999.

- is too closed
- will not open
- is too floppy
- is too open
- is too short
- is too stiff

Or, at either end of the eustachian tube, the system can

- be too closed
- be too open
- have abnormal pressure

More simply stated, dysfunction of the eustachian tube within its system can be summarized as follows: the tubal system is either *too closed* or *too open*, or there is *abnormal pressure* at either end.

The eustachian tube itself can be *too closed* when there is inflammation within the tube from infection (viral, bacterial) or allergy, but the tube can also be obstructed from external pressure, such as from tumor or adenoids (Figure 4-7). One of the most common findings in patients who have chronic and recurrent eustachian tube dysfunction is that the tube fails to open (*will not open*) during swallowing and even paradoxically constricts during swallowing activity, the etiology of which remains unknown at present (Figure 4-8). Also, studies have revealed that the tube can be *too floppy*, especially in infants and young children, which may be attributable to lack of stiffness of the tubal cartilage. Also, in infants and young children, the tube is *too short*, compared with older children and adults. The length and stiffness of the tube improve with advancing age (Figure 4-9). In some individuals, the tube can be *too open* and may even be patulous (*too open*) when the patient is not swallowing, which, in older individuals, may be attributable to increased tubal stiffness (ie, *too stiff*) (Figure 4-10).

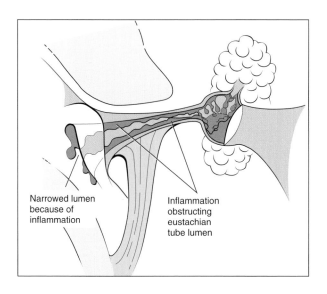

Narrowed lumen
because of
inflammation

Inflammation
obstructing
eustachian
tube lumen

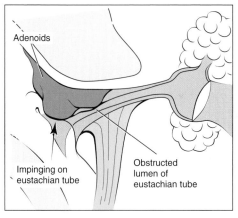

Adenoids

Impinging on
eustachian tube

Obstructed
lumen of
eustachian tube

Figure 4–7   Obstruction of the eustachian tube can be from inflammation or from extrinsic obstruction, such as from large adenoids. Reproduced from Bluestone CD. Conquering otitis media. Hamilton (ON): BC Decker; 1999.

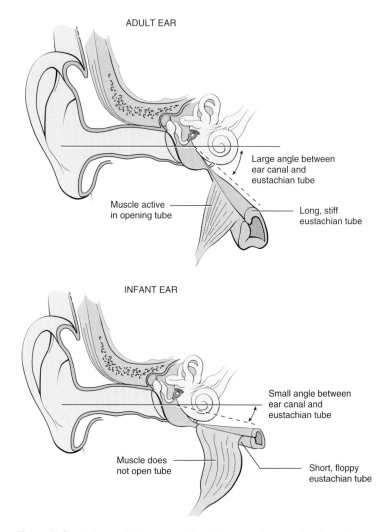

Figure 4–8 Failure of the eustachian tube opening mechanism. Reproduced from Bluestone CD. Conquering otitis media. Hamilton (ON): BC Decker; 1999.

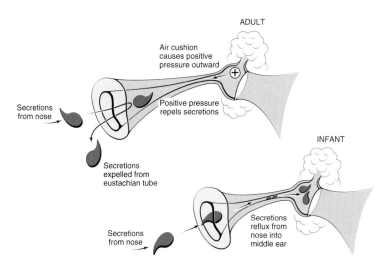

Figure 4–9 The eustachian tube is too short in infants and young children. Reproduced from Bluestone CD. Conquering otitis media. Hamilton (ON): BC Decker; 1999.

At either end of the tube, the system can be *too closed* even though the eustachian tube itself may have normal structure and function. At the middle ear end of the system, a mass, such as a cholesteatoma, tumor, or polyp, can block the opening into the eustachian tube. At the nasopharyngeal end of the

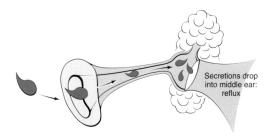

Figure 4–10 If the eustachian tube is too open, nasopharyngeal secretions can reflux into the middle ear. Reproduced from Bluestone CD. Conquering otitis media. Hamilton (ON): BC Decker; 1999.

tube, adenoids, tumor, or a foreign body (nasal packing) can obstruct the tubal opening.

In contrast to being too closed, the system can be *too open* at either end of the eustachian tube. At the middle ear end, a nonintact tympanic membrane is abnormal (eg, perforation or tympanostomy tube), and at the nasopharyngeal end, an open cleft palate is likewise abnormal (Figure 4-11). When there is high middle ear negative pressure, which occurs most commonly during an upper respiratory tract infection, the *abnormal pressure* can result in middle ear disease. At the nasopharyngeal end, swallowing when the nasal cavities are obstructed can result in abnormal nasopharyngeal pressures, which may then result in middle ear disease. This has been termed the "Toynbee phenomenon" (Figure 4-12). Also, ambient pressures can

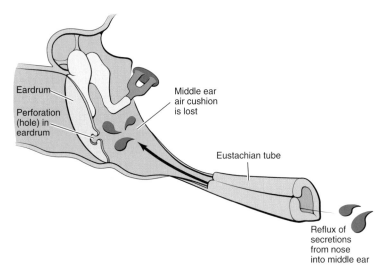

Eardrum

Perforation (hole) in eardrum

Middle ear air cushion is lost

Eustachian tube

Reflux of secretions from nose into middle ear

Figure 4–11 A nonintact tympanic membrane caused by a perforation or tympanostomy tube can promote reflux of secretions from the nasopharynx into the middle ear because the middle ear air cushion is impaired. Reproduced from Bluestone CD. Conquering otitis media. Hamilton (ON): BC Decker; 1999.

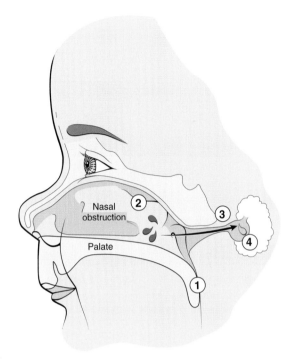

 Nasal obstruction

Palate

2

3

4

1

(1) Soft palate closes against nasopharynx during swallowing

(2) Pressure builds in nose

(3) Pressure in middle ear is less than pressure in nose

(4) Nasal secretions are forced into middle ear

Figure 4–12 Nasal obstruction can cause abnormal nasopharyngeal pressures, which can be related to eustachian tube dysfunction and middle ear disease. Reproduced from Bluestone CD. Conquering otitis media. Hamilton (ON): BC Decker; 1999.

be abnormal during unphysiologic activities, such as scuba diving, airplane flying, or hyperbaric treatments. Even diving into water during swimming, especially when an individual has an upper respiratory infection or allergic rhinitis, may result in an acute otitis media (Figure 4-13). Also, flying in air-

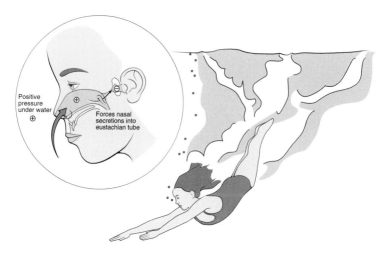

Figure 4–13 Diving into a swimming pool can cause acute otitis media when an upper respiratory infection is present. Reproduced from Bluestone CD. Conquering otitis media. Hamilton (ON): BC Decker; 1999.

planes can be the cause of barotrauma owing to abnormal pressures, especially during descent because the eustachian tube must open to equilibrate the pressure. If an individual has an upper respiratory infection and the eustachian tube is inflamed, middle ear effusion or even acute otitis media can develop (Figures 4-14 and 4-15).

Because infants have an immature eustachian tube function, they are prone to having problems during airplane flying during descent. Fortunately, they compensate by crying, which forces nasopharyngeal air into the middle ear to equilibrate the middle ear negative pressure (Figure 4-16).

A more precise and complete classification of eustachian tube function and dysfunction is shown in Table 4-1. For a more complete explanation and evidence, the reader is referred to Bluestone and Klein, 2003.

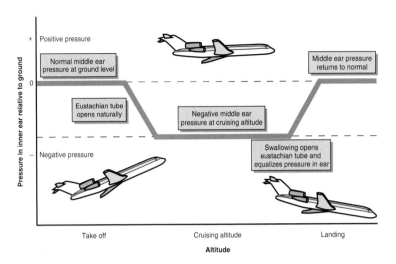

Figure 4–14 Explanation of how the normal eustachian tube and middle ear respond during airplane flying. Reproduced from Bluestone CD. Conquering otitis media. Hamilton (ON): BC Decker; 1999.

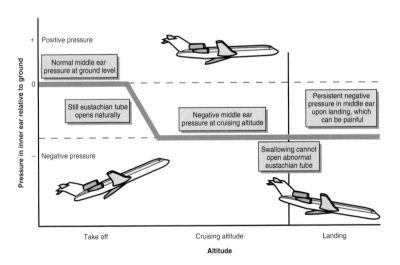

Figure 4–15 Explanation of how the abnormal eustachian tube and middle ear respond during airplane flying. Reproduced from Bluestone CD. Conquering otitis media. Hamilton (ON): BC Decker; 1999.

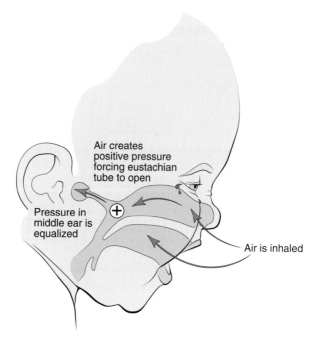

Figure 4–16 Most likely, infants cry during descent in airplanes to compensate for their lack of effective opening of the eustachian tube. Reproduced from Bluestone CD. Conquering otitis media. Hamilton (ON): BC Decker; 1999.

SEQUENCE OF EVENTS FOR OTITIS MEDIA

In a series of viral nasal challenge studies in adult volunteers, the following sequence occurs during an upper respiratory tract infection:

- history of eustachian tube dysfunction (ie, predisposition)
- upper respiratory viral infection
- eustachian tube obstruction
- high middle ear negative pressure
- middle ear effusion/infection

Table 4–1 Classification of Physiology and Pathophysiology of the Eustachian Tube

Physiology (Functions)
  Pressure regulation ("ventilatory function")
  Protection
    Anatomic
    Immunologic and mucociliary defense
  Clearance
    Mucociliary clearance
    Muscular clearance ("pumping action")
  Surface tension factors

Pathophysiology (Dysfunctions)
  Impairment of pressure regulation
    Anatomic obstruction
      Intraluminal
      Periluminal
      Peritubal
    Failure of opening mechanism ("functional obstruction")
  Loss of protective function
    Abnormal patency
    Short tube
    Abnormal gas pressures
      Intratympanic
      Nasopharyngeal
    Nonintact middle ear and mastoid
  Impairment of clearance
    Mucociliary
    Muscular

In subjects who had no history of middle ear disease, middle ear negative pressure—but no middle ear effusion—occurred during the viral challenge. In those who had a history of otitis media, middle ear effusion did occur and even a pneumococcal and viral acute otitis media (Buchman et al, 1995). Figure 4-17 also shows the most common sequence of events leading to a middle ear infection, and Figure 4-18 shows the development of otitis media with effusion, in which bacterial/viral infection is absent.

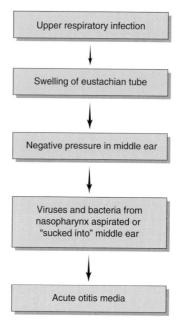

Figure 4–17 Sequence of events leading to acute otitis media. Reproduced from Bluestone CD. Conquering otitis media. Hamilton (ON): BC Decker; 1999.

WHY OTORRHEA OCCURS WITH OTITIS MEDIA

During an episode of acute otitis media, the tympanic membrane can rupture, causing acute otorrhea. In addition, when the tympanic membrane is not intact, owing to a chronic perforation or the presence of a tympanostomy tube, an attack of acute otitis media can result in acute otorrhea. If the acute otitis media and otorrhea persist, chronic otorrhea (ie, chronic suppurative otitis media) develops. When this occurs, the nonintact tympanic membrane is not protective as the normal middle ear air (gas) cushion is violated (ie, the middle ear is *too open*) and secretions from the nasopharynx "reflux" into the middle ear and then into the external ear canal. A nonintact

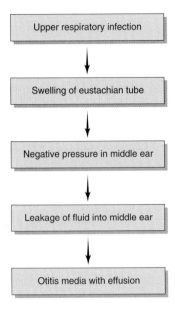

Figure 4–18 Sequence of events leading to otitis media with effusion. Reproduced from Bluestone CD. Conquering otitis media. Hamilton (ON): BC Decker; 1999.

tympanic membrane is also susceptible to contamination from the ear canal, such as from water (see Figure 4-11).

REFERENCES

Bluestone CD. Eustachian tube function and dysfunction. In: Rosenfeld RM, Bluestone CD, editors. Evidence-based otitis media. Hamilton (ON): BC Decker; 1999. p. 137–56.

Bluestone CD, Klein JO. Otitis media, atelectasis and eustachia tube dysfunction. In: Bluestone CD, Stool SE, Alper CM, et al, editors. Pediatric otolaryngology. 4th ed. Philadelphia: WB Saunders; 2003. p. 474–773.

Buchman CA, Doyle WJ, Skoner DP, et al. Influenza A virus-induced acute otitis media. J Infect Dis 1995;172:1348–51.

Casselbrant ML, Mandel EM, Fall PA, et al. The heritability of otitis media: a twin/triplet study. JAMA 1999;282:2125–30.

CHAPTER 5

MICROBIOLOGY

Viruses and bacteria can cause otitis media. Viruses can be isolated from about 25% of middle ear effusions of patients who have acute otitis media (Table 5-1).

The bacteria that cause acute otitis media are similar in children and adults (Bluestone et al, 1992; Celin et al, 1991). *Streptococcus pneumoniae* (40%), *Haemophilus influenzae* (25%), and *Moraxella catarrhalis* (12%) are the most common pathogens isolated. Group A β-hemolytic streptococcus and *Staphylococcus aureus* also cause acute otitis media in both children and adults but not as frequently as *S. pneumoniae* and *H. influenzae*. Contrary to earlier reports that found that gram-negative enteric bacteria cause about 20% of acute otitis media in neonates, a recent study reported that the same bacteria cause acute middle ear infections in infants younger than 2 months of age as when acute otitis media occurs in older infants and children (Turner et al, 2002). Respiratory viruses have been cultured from as many as 20% of acute effusions.

The percentage of *H. influenzae* that are β-lactamase-producing vary according to the community, but the rate is now about 25% in the United States (Dowell et al, 1998). Currently, most strains of *M. catarrhalis* produce β-lactamase. The rate of isolation of multidrug-resistant *S. pneumoniae* is increasing in the United States. At the Children's Hospital of Pittsburgh—a

Table 5–1   Viruses Found in Middle Ear Effusions
Respiratory syncytial virus
Rhinovirus
Influenza virus
Adenovirus
Parainfluenza viruses
Enteroviruses

tertiary referral center—our rate increased from approximately 10% in 1988 to over 40% in 2002, and more than half of these strains were highly resistant. Most likely, the rate is lower in community practices. Failure of an antibiotic to eradicate these resistant organisms has been shown to be more likely associated with a clinical treatment failure than when the drug sterilizes the middle ear infection (Dagan et al, 1996). Increased risk for development of antimicrobial-resistant pneumococci has been attributed to low-dose and prolonged treatment with β-lactam antimicrobial agents, recent exposure to antibiotics, child day-

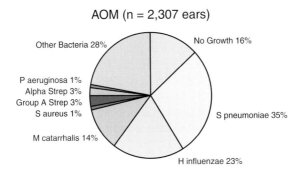

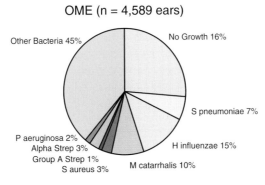

Figure 5–1 Distribution of middle ear isolates from ears of infants and children who had acute otitis media and otitis media with effusion. Reproduced with permission from Bluestone CD, Stool SE, Alper CM, et al, editors. Pediatric otolaryngology. 4th ed. Philadelphia: WB Saunders; 2003.

care attendance, age less than 2 years, otitis-prone infants, and winter season (Guillemot et al, 1998; Negri et al, 1994).

Bacteria can be isolated from approximately two-thirds of middle ears with otitis media with effusion, but only one-third are considered to be possibly pathogenic, for example, *H. influenzae*, *M. catarrhalis*, and *S. pneumoniae* (Bluestone et al, 1992). However, polymerase chain reaction has identified these organisms in a much larger percentage (Post et al, l995; Rayner et al, 1998).

Figure 5-1 shows the distribution of middle ear isolates from ears with acute otitis media and otitis media with effusion.

REFERENCES

Bluestone CD, Stephenson JS, Martin LM. Ten-year review of otitis media pathogens. Pediatr Infect Dis J 1992;11:S7–11.

Celin SE, Bluestone CD, Stephenson J, et al. Bacteriology of acute otitis media in adults. JAMA 1991;266:2249–52.

Dagan R, Abramson O, Leibovitz E, et al. Impaired bacteriologic response to oral cephalosporins in acute otitis media caused by pneumococci with intermediate resistant to penicillin. Pediatr Infect Dis J 1996;15:980–5.

Dowell SF, Marcy SM, Phillips WR, et al. Otitis media—principles of judicious use of antimicrobial agents. In: Dowell SF, editor. Principles of judicious use of antimicrobial agents for pediatric upper respiratory tract infections. Pediatrics 1998;101 Suppl:165–6.

Guillemot D, Carbon C, Balkau B, et al. Low dosage and long treatment duration of beta lactam: risk factors for carriage of penicillin-resistant *Streptococcus pneumoniae*. JAMA 1998;279:365–70.

Negri MC, Morosini MI, Loza E, Baquero F. In vitro selective antibiotic concentrations of beta-lactams for penicillin-resistant *Streptococcus pneumoniae* populations. Antimicrob Agents Chemother 1994;38:122–5.

Post JC, Preston RA, Aul JJ, et al. Molecular analysis of bacterial pathogens in otitis media with effusion. JAMA 1995;273:1598–604.

Rayner MG, Zhang Y, Gorry MC, et al. Evidence of bacterial metabolic activity in culture-negative otitis media with effusion. JAMA 1998; 279:296–9.

Turner D, Leibovitz E, Aran A, et al. Acute otitis media in infants younger than two months of age: microbiology, clinical presentation and therapeutic approach. Pediatr Infect Dis J 2002;21:669–74.

CHAPTER 6

DIAGNOSIS

It is important to distinguish between acute otitis media and otitis media with effusion because management options will depend on which disease entity is present. The most important diagnostic method, in addition to the medical history, is assessment of the appearance and mobility of the tympanic membrane, which includes pneumatic otoscopy (Figure 6-1).

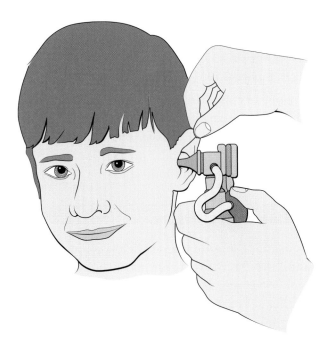

Figure 6–1 The pneumatic otoscope should be used with the largest speculum that fits comfortably into the patient's ear canal meatus; insertion too deeply will elicit pain. Gentle pressure should be used initially to determine if the tympanic moves freely in and out. If it does not, then more pressure can be applied. Reproduced from Bluestone CD. Conquering otitis media. Hamilton (ON): BC Decker; 1999.

ACUTE OTITIS MEDIA

Acute otitis media is characterized by the rapid onset of signs and symptoms of infection in the middle ear. Synonyms such as *acute suppurative* or *purulent otitis media* are also in common use. One or more of the following symptoms are present: otalgia (or pulling of the ear in the young infant), fever, or irritability of recent onset. The tympanic membrane is full or bulging and opaque and has limited or no mobility to pneumatic otoscopy. The acute onset of ear pain, fever, and a purulent discharge (otorrhea) through a perforation of the tympanic membrane or tympanostomy tube would also be evidence of acute otitis media. The distinction between acute severe otitis media and infections that are less severe depends on the degree of fever and the severity of the otalgia, as well as the presence or absence of a bulging tympanic membrane.

Following an episode of acute otitis media, the middle ear may have fluid that remains for weeks to months and has been termed *persistent middle ear effusion*. The signs and symptoms associated with persistent middle ear effusion are usually the same as otitis media with effusion, which are described below.

OTITIS MEDIA WITH EFFUSION

Otitis media with effusion is a relatively asymptomatic middle ear effusion that has many synonyms, such as *secretory*, *nonsuppurative*, or *serous otitis media*. Pneumatic otoscopy frequently reveals either a retracted or concave tympanic membrane, which has limited or absent mobility. However, fullness or even bulging may be visualized. In addition, an air-fluid level or bubbles, or both, may be observed through a translucent tympanic membrane.

The most important distinction between acute otitis media and otitis media with effusion is that the signs and symptoms of acute infection such as otalgia and fever are lacking in otitis media with effusion, but middle ear effusion occurs in both, and hearing loss is usually present in both conditions (Table 6-1). Figure 6-2 shows some examples of tympanic membranes when the eardrum is normal and abnormal when visualized using the pneumatic otoscope.

TYMPANOCENTESIS

The clinician can perform an aspiration of the middle ear fluid when the diagnosis of acute otitis media is in doubt or when determination of the etiologic agent is desirable. If he or she is not skilled in this procedure, the patient can be referred to an otolaryngologist (Bluestone and Klein, 2001). Tympanocentesis is an increasingly important diagnostic procedure with the emergence of antibiotic-resistant bacterial organisms causing otitis media, such as β-lactamase-producing *Haemophilus influenzae* and *Moraxella catarrhalis*, and the more recent troublesome rise in penicillin and multidrug-resistant pneumococcus during the last decade (Spika et al, 1991; Welby et al, 1994) (Table 6-2). Also, if otorrhea is present with the acute otitis media, a culture can be obtained from the drainage.

	Otalgia, Fever, Irritability	Middle Ear Effusion	Opaque Drum	Retracted Drum	Impaired Mobility of drum	Hearing Loss
Table 6–1 Diagnostic Similarities and Differences between Acute Otitis Media and Otitis Media with Effusion						
Acute otitis media	Usually present	Present	Present	Absent	Present	Present
Otitis media with effusion	Absent	Present (air-fluid level, bubbles)	May be present	Usually present	Present	Usually present

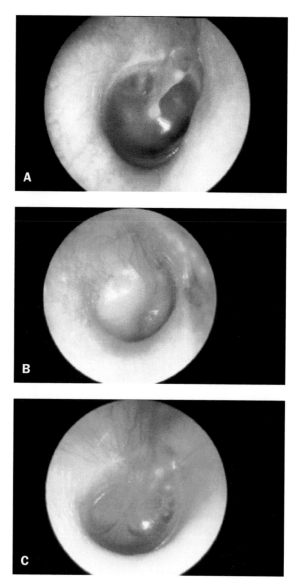

Figure 6–2 Examples of tympanic membranes when the eardrum is normal and abnormal when visualized using the pneumatic otoscope. A, normal; B, acute otitis media; C, otitis media with effusion. Reproduced from Bluestone CD. Conquering otitis media. Hamilton (ON): BC Decker; 1999.

Table 6–2 Recommended Indications for Tympanocentesis (Myringotomy)
Otitis media in patients who have severe otalgia, are seriously ill, or appear toxic
Unsatisfactory response to antimicrobial therapy
Onset of otitis media in a patient who is receiving antimicrobial therapy
Otitis media associated with a confirmed or potential suppurative complication
Otitis media in a newborn, sick neonate, or immunologically deficient patient, any of whom might harbor an unusual organism

Tympanocentesis is a needle aspiration of middle ear fluid through the membrane that can be performed using an 18-gauge spinal needle attached to a tuberculin syringe. In contrast, a myringotomy (performed using a myringotomy knife) is a drainage procedure of the middle ear that is indicated when

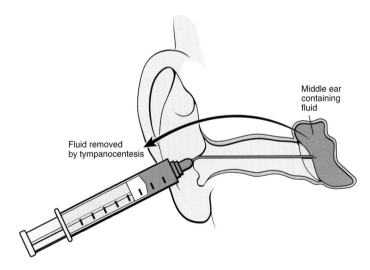

Figure 6–3 Tympanocentesis can be performed using a needle attached to a syringe. Reproduced from Bluestone CD. Conquering otitis media. Hamilton (ON): BC Decker; 1999.

there is acute, severe otalgia or a suppurative complication of otitis media or whenever a tympanocentesis is performed to provide more adequate drainage of the middle ear and mastoid (Figure 6-3).

Tympanometry is helpful in confirming that a middle ear effusion is present but does not distinguish between acute otitis media and otitis media with effusion. This is best accomplished by the history and physical examination that includes the otoscopic appearance and mobility of the tympanic membrane using the pneumatic otoscope. Assessments of hearing are not diagnostic of a middle ear effusion but can be helpful in management decisions.

REFERENCES

Bluestone CD. Eustachian tube function and dysfunction. In: Rosenfeld RM, Bluestone CD, editors. Evidence-based otitis media. Hamilton (ON): BC Decker; 1999. p. 137–56.

Bluestone CD, Klein JO. Otitis media in infants and children. 3rd ed. Philadelphia: WB Saunders; 2001.

Spika JS, Facklam RR, Plikaytis BD, Oxtoby MT. Antimicrobial resistance of *Streptococcus pneumoniae* in the United States, 1979-1987. The pneumococcal surveillance working group. J Infect Dis 1991; 163:1273–8.

Welby PL, Keller DS, Cromien JL, et al. Resistance to penicillin and no-beta-lactam antibiotics of *Streptococcus pneumoniae* at a children's hospital. Pediatr Infect Dis J 1994;13:281–7.

CHAPTER 7

MANAGEMENT

As emphasized in Chapter 6, "Diagnosis," it is important to make the most accurate diagnosis possible between acute otitis media and otitis media with effusion because management decisions will differ.

ACUTE OTITIS MEDIA

Once the diagnosis of acute otitis media is confirmed, the clinician must make several management decisions. Some are controversial.

To Treat or Not To Treat?

With the possibility of increasing the problem of drug-resistant bacterial pathogens, some clinicians, especially in some European countries and a few in the United States, question the need for antimicrobial therapy in all patients for treatment of acute otitis media (Culpepper and Froom, 1997; van Buchem et al, 1981). However, most experts in the United States today agree that acute otitis media should be actively treated with an antimicrobial agent. Some of the compelling evidence for their use is listed in Table 7-1. We addressed this issue in a large clinical trial in Pittsburgh, in which we found that subjects who had episodes of "severe" acute otitis media and who had been randomized to receive myringotomy without antibiotics had statistically more initial treatment failures than those children who received an antimicrobial agent, with or without the adjunctive use of a myringotomy. Myringotomy is not necessary for routine treatment of uncomplicated attacks (Kaleida et al, 1991) but is indicated for the indications listed in Table 6-2. As part of that trial, another group of children who had "nonsevere" acute otitis media were randomized to either antibiotic

Table 7–1 Evidence That Antimicrobial Agents Are Indicated for Treatment of Acute Otitis Media
Compared with placebo (or no drug), antimicrobials:
• Sterilize the middle ear effusion (Howie and Ploussard, 1972).
• Result in earlier resolution of symptoms of acute infection (Rosenfeld et al, 1994).
• Shorten time with middle ear effusion (hearing loss) (Kaleida et al, 1991).
• Dramatically decrease suppurative complications (Lahikainen, 1953; Rudberg, 1954).

or placebo. Subjects in the placebo group also had more treatment failures and more time with middle ear effusion compared with those in the antibiotic group.

The Centers for Disease Control and Prevention and the American Academy of Pediatrics have reaffirmed the recommendation to treat all confirmed cases (Dowell et al, 1998). In the Netherlands, in which antimicrobials are withheld pending possible spontaneous resolution of the acute symptoms, a second visit to the physician is required. If observation is unsuccessful, antibiotic treatment is instituted. In addition to the established efficacy of antimicrobial treatment—the antibiotic resistance problem notwithstanding—instituting active treatment will result in a return visit to the clinician only for antibiotic treatment failures and routine follow-up, which appears to be more cost-effective (related to physician visits) than withholding a drug such as amoxicillin. Approximately 20% fail to improve without the benefit of antimicrobial therapy, whereas only about 5% fail on amoxicillin (Mandel et al, 1993; Rosenfeld et al, 1994).

A recent review by Hendley (2002) recommends that the clinician distinguish between those patients who have bulging tympanic membranes and those who do not, with immediate treatment for those whose drums are bulging and delayed treatment for children whose drums are not. This recommendation is arbitrary and without support from randomized clinical trials. Until such trials are available, there is now sufficient evidence of the safety and efficacy of antibiotic therapy to warrant treatment in all patients with a moderate to severe acute middle ear infection. However, for children, especially those above age 2 years, who have mild acute otitis media, antibiotics may be delayed for 48 to 72 hours to determine if spontaneous resolution of symptoms occurs because spontaneous resolution is more likely when the infection is nonsevere. As mentioned previously, it is important to distinguish acute otitis media from the relatively asymptomatic otitis media with effusion because the latter disease is usually not treated unless the effusion becomes chronic.

Which Antimicrobial Agent?

Amoxicillin is currently recommended for initial routine empiric therapy of uncomplicated acute otitis media. It is active both in vitro and in vivo against most strains of *Streptococcus pneumoniae* and *Haemophilus influenzae* and is relatively inexpensive in the United States (Berman et al, 1997; Dowell et al, 1998). If the patient is allergic to the penicillins, one of the cephalosporins (eg, cefuroxime, cefpodoxime, or cefdinir) could be used if the patient does not have hypersensitivity to these agents and does not have an immediate hypersensitivity reaction to the penicillins. If the patient is allergic to both the penicillins and the cephalosporins, then one of the macrolides or erythromycin-sulfamethoxazole can be given.

Trimethoprim-sulfamethoxazole is not a desirable alternative because it has had an unacceptable safety record. *S. pneumoniae* isolates are increasing in resistance rates to the macrolides (Hyde et al, 2001). A single parenteral dose of ceftriaxone is the most recent antimicrobial agent approved for treatment. It is particularly useful for those ambulatory patients when compliance with the oral agents is uncertain, when convenience of one parenterally administered dose is desirable, or in those infants and children who have severe otitis media (Barnett et al, 1997).

Table 7-2 provides a list of the approved antimicrobial agents with their recommended dosing schedules. Empiric use of such agents as the tetracyclines, penicillin V, erythromycin, or cephalexin is not recommended as monotherapy. The quinolones, such as ciprofloxacin, are not indicated in children below 17 years of age, and efficacy of these antimicrobial agents has not been reported in adults with acute otitis media.

The traditional 10- to 14-day course of therapy is usually recommended, but there has been a recent proposal to shorten the course to 5 to 7 days in certain children above the age of 2 years in an effort to reduce antibiotic use (Dowell et al, 1998; Paradise, 1997). High-dose amoxicillin, for a short course, has been shown to reduce the rate of resistant pneumococcal nasopharyngeal carriage (Schrag et al, 2001).

Treatment Failures

Most attacks of acute otitis media improve significantly within 48 to 72 hours when appropriate antimicrobial therapy is administered. If signs and symptoms of infection progress despite this treatment, that is, treatment failure, the patient should be re-evaluated within 24 hours because a suppurative complication or a concurrent serious infection may have developed (eg, an infant may have meningitis). Persistent or recurrent pain or fever, or both, during treatment (also a treatment failure) would signal the need for tympanocentesis and myringotomy (for Gram stain, culture, and susceptibility testing), selection of another antimicrobial agent, or both (see Chapter 6, "Diagnosis"). Selection of an antibiotic at this stage would depend on the results of the culture and susceptibility

Table 7–2   Antimicrobial Agents Available for Treatment of Otitis Media*

Antimicrobial Agents	Dosing Schedule
Penicillins	
Amoxicillin[†]	40 mg/kg/d in 3 doses
Amoxicillin-clavulanate	45 mg/kg/d in 2 doses
(Augmentin ES)	90 mg/kg/d in 2 doses
Cephalosporins	
Cefaclor (Ceclor)	40 mg/kg/d in 2 or 3 doses
Loracarbef (Lorabid)	30 mg/kg/d in 2 doses
Cefuroxime-axetil (Ceftin)	30 mg/kg/d in 2 doses
Cefpodoxime (Vantin)	10 mg/kg/d once daily
Cefixime (Suprax)	8 mg/kg/d once daily or in 2 doses
Ceftibuten (Cedax)	8 mg/kg/d once daily or in 2 doses
Cefdinir (Omnicef)	14 mg/kg/d once daily
Ceftriaxone (Rocephin)[‡]	50 mg/kg in one parenteral dose
Macrolides	
Erythromycin	50 mg/kg/d in 4 doses
Clarithromycin (Biaxin)	7.5 mg/kg/d in 2 doses
Azithromycin (Zithromax)	10 mg/kg day 1, 5 mg/kg days 2–5
Sulfa Combinations	
Erythromycin-sulfisoxazole (Pediazole)	50 mg/kg/d (erythromycin); 150 mg/kg/d in 4 doses (sulfisoxazole)
Trimethoprim-sulfamethoxazole (Bactrim, Septra)	8 mg/kg/d (trimethoprim); 40 mg/kg/d in 2 doses (sulfamethoxazole)
Ototopical Agents	
Ofloxacin otic solution 0.3% (Floxin Otic)	5–10 drops in 2 doses
Ciprofloxacin-dexamethasone (CiproDex)[§]	

*Includes the oral agents and one parenteral drug available for treatment on an ambulatory basis, whereas there are other parenteral antimicrobial agents effective for treatment of otitis media, usually on an inpatient basis; also, two ototopical agents are listed.

†Double dose of amoxicillin when antibiotic-resistant pneumococcus is suspected or isolated.

‡Available only in parenteral form.

§US Food and Drug Administration approval pending as of February 2003.

testing. If amoxicillin was initially administered, then one of the alternative antimicrobial agents to this drug that covers β-lactamase-producing bacteria as well as resistant *S. pneumoniae* should be selected. This would be reasonable as empiric therapy until the results of the culture are available or if a culture is not obtained (see Table 7-2).

Acute Otitis Media with Perforation and Otorrhea

When an episode of acute otitis media occurs, the tympanic membrane may rupture and otorrhea may develop. Even though there are no clinical trials to demonstrate effectiveness, an ototopical agent should be prescribed in addition to the systemic antimicrobial agent. The rationale for the addition of an ototopical antimicrobial agent (with or without a corticosteroid) is not only to treat the middle ear and external auditory canal infection but also to prevent a secondary middle ear (mastoid) infection owing to bacteria such as *Pseudomonas* or *Staphylococcus aureus*, which can become chronic (ie, chronic suppurative otitis media). It should be noted that chronic otorrhea starts with acute otorrhea; thus, if the acute infection is cured, chronic infection will be prevented (see Chapter 8, "Complications and Sequelae," in the section on chronic suppurative otitis media).

The appropriate agent should be effective against the common pathogenic bacterial organisms that cause acute otitis media and should not be ototoxic. Today, the otopical agents that have been shown to be safe and effective when acute otitis media occurs and when a tympanostomy tube is in place appear to be a reasonable treatment option to use for this indication. Ofloxacin otic solution 0.3% (Floxin Otic) and ciprofloxacin-dexamethasone (CiproDex) are recommended, but the latter appears to be more effective when acute otorrhea occurs through a tympanostomy tube (Dohar et al, 1996, 1999; Roland, 2001).

Follow-up Visits and Persistent Middle Ear Effusion

Patients should be re-examined at the end of the course of antibiotic therapy if they still have any signs or symptoms of acute infection because further evaluation and therapy may be indicated. However, the presence of effusion after a trial of an antimicrobial agent occurs in many infants and children, and when it is asymptomatic, the patient does *not* require further treatment with an antimicrobial agent unless the effusion progresses to the chronic stage (Dowell et al, 1998; Stool et al, 1994). Persistence of middle ear effusion for weeks to months after the onset of acute otitis media was frequent in Boston children (Teele et al, 1983): 70% of children still had effusion at 2 weeks, 40% had effusion at 1 month, 20% had effusion at 2 months, and 10% had effusion at 3 months. Similar rates of persistent middle ear effusion after an episode of acute otitis media have been noted in recent studies from other centers, with the exception of one of our studies in Pittsburgh. We included recurrent acute otitis media for this outcome, which occurred in 50% of subjects during the following 3 months. The point prevalence of persistent and recurrent middle ear effusion was 40% after 30 days and 23% at 90 days after the onset of the initial attack (Kaleida et al, 1987).

If the child is not a treatment failure at the end of treatment, the first follow-up visit can safely be delayed. Mandel and colleagues (1995) conducted a clinical trial in children in which 20-day therapy was compared with the traditional 10-day course. We recommended having children who were asymptomatic return for their first follow-up visit in 4 weeks because further treatment with antimicrobial therapy immediately after 10-day treatment in the trial provided no long-term advantage. This recommendation represents a significant cost saving. If an asymptomatic effusion fails to spontaneously resolve, factors that would be important in deciding to treat or not to treat this stage of the disease are similar to those described in the section on otitis media with effusion.

RECURRENT ACUTE OTITIS MEDIA

If attacks of acute otitis media are frequent and close together (eg, three or more episodes in 6 months or four or more attacks in 12 months, with one being recent), prevention is desirable. Such a patient requires further evaluation. Several avenues of investigation are open: a search for respiratory allergy, roentgenograms (or imaging) of the paranasal sinuses may reveal sinusitis, immunologic studies may be of value if other organs are involved (ie, the lungs), an evaluation of immune function for children over age 5 years might be helpful even if recurrent or chronic ear disease is the only apparent problem, and a more complete evaluation of the head and neck may uncover a tumor, especially in adolescents and adults. If none of the above conditions is present, then one or more of the popular methods of prevention may be attempted.

Nonsurgical Options

Parents can be informed about the possible risk factors described in Chapter 3, "Epidemiology," in an attempt to reduce the attack rate of acute otitis media and the factors that can be introduced to reduce the rate, such as breast-feeding in place of the bottle, reducing daycare attendance (the greater the number of children, the higher the frequency of attacks), elimination of smoking in the household, and elimination of pacifiers past the age of 1 year (Dowell et al, 1998). The new conjugate pneumococcal vaccine, Prevnar, is now administered to all infants to prevent invasive pneumococcal disease, and the clinician should confirm that this vaccine was received (Pelton and Klein, 2002). Even though the reduction in the attack rate of acute otitis media was relatively modest in the clinical trials, there was a reduction in episodes in patients who had recurrent acute otitis media and the number of children who required tympanostomy tubes in those who received the conjugate vaccine (Bluestone, 2001; Fireman et al, 2003). Also, any child who has frequently had recurrent acute otitis media, irrespective of age, might benefit from either the conjugate or the older polysaccharide vaccine, depending on age. Administration of the influenza vaccine may also benefit in reducing the attack rate (Bluestone and Klein, 2003).

Antimicrobial prophylaxis for the prevention of recurrent acute otitis media has been demonstrated to be effective (Williams et al, 1993). We recommend amoxicillin, 20 mg/kg in one dose (given at bedtime), which has been shown to be safe and effective (Casselbrant et al, 1992). If the child is allergic to the penicillins, a daily dose of sulfisoxazole 50 mg/kg may be substituted. There is now some evidence that prophylaxis with amoxicillin is more likely to be associated with the colonization of β-lactamase-producing bacteria and resistant pneumococcus than sulfisoxazole (Dowell et al, 1998). However, the established safety of long-term prophylaxis with the penicillins (ie, experience with prevention of streptococcal throat infection in patients with rheumatic heart disease) must be weighed against the possible adverse reactions associated with prolonged administration of the sulfas (eg, trimethoprim and sulfamethoxazole). The prophylactic regimen should be continued during the respiratory seasons. It is important to stress that instituting antimicrobial prophylaxis is inappropriate if long-standing chronic middle ear effusion is present. When this occurs, the patient should be managed as described in the section on otitis media with effusion.

Surgical Options

With the growing evidence that long-term antimicrobial prophylaxis is associated with the emergence of resistant *Pneumo-*

coccus in infants and young children, a more desirable option is tympanostomy tube placement (Bluestone et al, 1994; Dowell et al, 1998). This operation has been shown to be effective for prevention of otitis media, compared with placebo, over a 2-year period (Casselbrant et al, 1992). Sequelae of tympanostomy tubes are common but are generally transient (such as when otorrhea develops) or cosmetic, for example, myringosclerosis (see the section on otitis media with effusion) (Kay et al, 2001) (Figures 7-1 and 7-2).

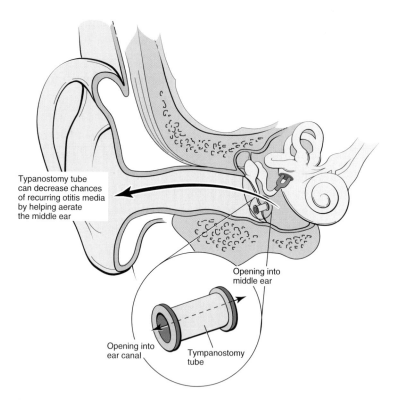

Figure 7-1 Artist's drawing of tympanostomy tube placement. Reproduced from Bluestone CD. Conquering otitis media. Hamilton (ON): BC Decker; 1999.

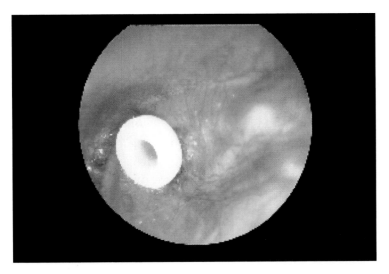

Figure 7–2 Otoscopic view of a tympanostomy tube. Reproduced from Bluestone CD. Conquering otitis media. Hamilton (ON): BC Decker; 1999.

Adenoidectomy, with or without tonsillectomy, is frequently advocated for the prevention of recurrent acute otitis media, but only one randomized, controlled study has been reported that has shown the efficacy of adenoidectomy, albeit limited, for this condition. Paradise and coworkers (1990) did demonstrate a significant difference in the attack rate of acute otitis media in children who had been randomized to receive adenoidectomy compared with those who did not receive this operation. All subjects in this clinical trial had at least one tympanostomy tube insertion prior to random assignment. A subsequent trial by our group failed to show efficacy when subjects had not had prior tympanostomy tube insertions, that is, less severely affected children (Paradise et al, 1999). As a note of caution, adenoidectomy in infants should only be recommended selectively—such as in those who also have severe nasal obstruction owing to obstructive adenoids—because the operation carries some degree of increased risk in this age group (Figure 7-3).

Which Management Option Today?

The decision today should be between recommending the nonsurgical methods of prevention—eliminating day care, passive smoking, and pacifiers; administering vaccines; or placing the child on an antibiotic in a prophylactic dose—and surgery. Citing the increasing drug-resistance problem, Paradise and

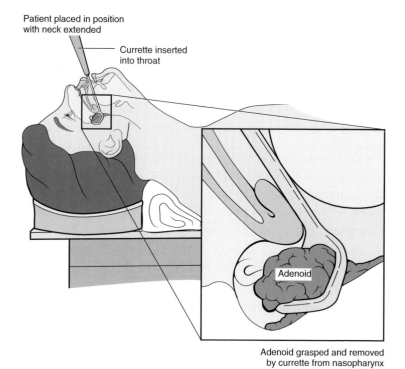

Patient placed in position with neck extended

Currette inserted into throat

Adenoid

Adenoid grasped and removed by currette from nasopharynx

Figure 7–3 The method to remove adenoids is shown in which a curette is used. Adenoids can also be removed by electrocoagulation. Reproduced from Bluestone CD. Conquering otitis media. Hamilton (ON): BC Decker; 1999.

colleagues (1995) recently advised against antibiotic prophylaxis and recommended this option only on an individualized basis. Currently, we recommend insertion of tympanostomy tubes as a more rational alternative to a long-term course of antibiotic prophylaxis. Adenoidectomy is also an option in selected cases.

OTITIS MEDIA WITH EFFUSION

Similar to treatment of acute otitis media, management of patients with otitis media with effusion is currently the subject of considerable debate. However, we now have enough evidence-based information to make some of the important decisions regarding treatment or no treatment and which therapeutic options are effective and which ones are not (Rosenfeld and Bluestone, 1999).

To Treat or Not To Treat?

Otitis media with effusion in most children will resolve without active treatment in 2 or 3 months (Casselbrant et al, 1985), but treatment may be indicated in some children because of the possible complications and sequelae associated with this condition. Because impairment of hearing of some degree usually accompanies a middle ear effusion (Fria et al, 1985), treatment may be warranted when long-standing hearing loss is present. Although the significance of this hearing loss is still uncertain, such a loss may impair cognitive and language function and result in disturbances in psychosocial adjustment (Teele et al, 1989). Important factors that should be considered when deciding to treat (and which treatment) or not to treat are listed in Table 7-3. The most compelling indications would be progression of the disease into the chronic stage (Dowell et al, 1998; Stool et al, 1994). Similar to a patient who has had recurrent acute otitis media, a thorough search for an underly-

Table 7–3   Factors To Be Considered on an Individual Basis Favoring Treatment with Antimicrobial Agents for Otitis Media with Effusion

Significant associated conductive hearing loss owing to the effusion

Occurrence in young infants because they are unable to communicate about their symptoms and may have suppurative disease

An associated acute suppurative upper respiratory tract infection

Concurrent permanent conductive/sensorineural hearing loss

Presence of speech/language delay associated with effusion and hearing loss

Balance disturbance such as clumsiness or falling

Alterations of the tympanic membrane, such as a retraction pocket

Middle ear changes, such as adhesive otitis media or ossicular involvement

Previous surgery for otitis media, eg, tympanostomy tube placement or adenoidectomy

Frequently recurring episodes

Effusion that persists for 3 months or longer, ie, chronic otitis media with effusion, prior to consideration for tympanostomy tube placement

ing etiology should be attempted before initiating a nonsurgical or surgical method of management of patients with frequently recurrent or chronic effusions.

Nonsurgical Treatment Options

If active treatment is elected, options are limited. Even though a combination of an oral decongestant and antihistamine was thought to be effective—and was widely used—in the past, two Pittsburgh studies that involved over 1,000 infants and children failed to demonstrate their efficacy in eliminating middle ear effusion (Cantekin et al, 1983; Mandel et al, 1987). Despite the apparent efficacy of systemic corticosteroid therapy in clinical trials (Rosenfeld et al, 1991), the official government guideline found the risks of this option in children to outweigh its possible benefits (Stool et al, 1994). To date, no clinical trials have been reported that have tested the efficacy of topical nasal corticosteroid treatment, immunotherapy, and control of allergy in children who have nasal allergy and middle ear disease. Nevertheless, this method of management seems reasonable in children who frequently have recurrent or chronic otitis media with effusion and evidence of upper respiratory allergy. Inflation of the eustachian tube/middle ear using Politzer's method or Valsalva's maneuver has been advocated for more than a century for this condition. However, a randomized, controlled trial by Chan and Bluestone (1989) found a lack of efficacy of middle ear inflation for chronic effusion; therefore, it is not recommended in children, and efficacy in adults remains uncertain. Inflation may be effective for all age groups for the management of middle ear effusion that follows barotrauma, such as after air travel or scuba diving.

Of all of the medical treatments that have been advocated, a trial of an antimicrobial agent would appear to be most appropriate in those children who have not received an antibiotic recently. A meta-analysis of the effect of antimicrobial agents in the treatment of otitis media with effusion was reported by Rosenfeld and Post (1992) that confirmed their efficacy, particularly when the effusion was chronic. Two other meta-analyses also verified their short-term effect, but, as expected, there was no long-term efficacy (Stool et al, 1994; Williams et al, 1993). Other strategies, such as antimicrobial prophylaxis (Mandel et al, 1996) or surgery, are required for long-term control because the disease frequently recurs owing to repeated exposure to upper respiratory tract infections.

As in acute otitis media, amoxicillin is a reasonable choice for treating otitis media with effusion. Our clinical trial demonstrated its efficacy, albeit limited, in the 518 infants and children who participated in the study (Mandel et al, 1987). Other antimicrobial agents have also been recommended, but none have been reported to be more effective than amoxicillin at this time. Cefaclor, erythromycin-sulfisoxazole, and ceftibuten have been shown to be equal or inferior to amoxicillin (Mandel et al, 1991, 1996). In a recently reported trial, the efficacy of a longer than 10-day course of amoxicillin was no more effective than the standard 10-day course for chronic otitis media with effusion (Mandel et al, 2002). Prolonging antimicrobial treatment for longer than 2 weeks is excessive and not recommended, especially with our current antibiotic-resistance problem.

When the effusion is chronic, surgical intervention should be considered, especially when antimicrobial therapy fails. Even though the official guideline from the government has recommended either antimicrobial therapy or tympanostomy tube insertion for bilateral chronic effusions (ie, 3 to 4 months duration) associated with hearing loss (Stool et al, 1994), a trial of amoxicillin therapy seems the most rational, regardless of the level of hearing (Bluestone et al, 1994). Indeed, a recent trial of antibiotic therapy conducted in the Netherlands by primary care physicians, who normally reserve these drugs for only severe acute otitis media, was found to be so effective that they recommended a course prior to referral of the patient to an otolaryngologist for surgery (van Balen et al, 1996).

Surgical Options

Myringotomy with tympanostomy tube placement or adenoidectomy and myringotomy, with and without tube insertion, has been demonstrated to be effective in children with chronic effusions that are unresponsive to a trial of antibiotics. Our two Pittsburgh clinical trials showed that tympanostomy tube insertion was more effective than myringotomy without tube insertion or no surgery (ie, controls) for chronic effusions (Mandel et al, 1989, 1992). Our recommendations for insertion of tympanostomy tubes in children are listed in Table 7-4.

Table 7–4   Recommended Indications for Tympanostomy Tube Insertion

Chronic otitis media with effusion, unresponsive to antimicrobial treatment, that has persisted for at least 3 months when bilateral or 6 months when unilateral

Recurrent acute otitis media, especially when antimicrobial prophylaxis fails. Minimum frequency for tube insertion would be three or more episodes during the previous 6 months or four or more attacks during the previous year, with one being recent.

Recurrent episodes of otitis media with effusion in which the duration of each episode does not meet criteria for chronic disease, but cumulative duration is considered excessive, such as 6 of the previous 12 months

Suppurative complication is suspected or present. Insertion of a tympanostomy tube at the time of tympanocentesis/myringotomy can provide more prolonged drainage and aeration of the middle ear–mastoid.

Eustachian tube dysfunction (even without middle ear effusion) when the patient has persistent/recurrent signs and symptoms not relieved by medical treatment options or at the time of reconstructive middle ear surgery. Signs and symptoms include hearing loss (usually fluctuating), dysequilibrium/vertigo, tinnitus, autophony, and severe retraction pocket.

Barotrauma, such as following airplane flying or hyperbaric chamber treatment, especially for prevention of recurrent episodes

Most permanent tympanostomy tubes last longer than the traditional grommet tubes, as the name implies. Grommet tubes usually remain in place and are functional for about 12 to 18 months, whereas the permanent tubes frequently last for a few years. The most compelling indication to insert a permanent tympanostomy tube is when eustachian tube dysfunction is chronic and is usually associated with chronic otitis media with recurrent effusion, and the patient has failed to improve after several sets of the standard grommet tubes (Figure 7-4).

Although there are evidenced-based indications for placement of tympanostomy tubes, there are known complications and sequelae. These include myringosclerosis and scarring and

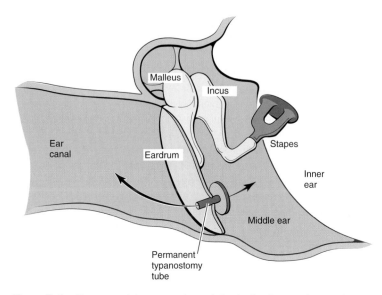

Figure 7–4 Permanent tympanostomy tube in the tympanic membrane. Reproduced from Bluestone CD. Conquering otitis media. Hamilton (ON): BC Decker; 1999.

thinning of the eardrum (dimeric membrane) (Figure 7-5) (Kay et al, 2001). The latter sequela may lead to, albeit rarely, a retraction pocket that can develop into an iatrogenic cholesteatoma. The most common complication is acute post-tympanostomy acute otitis media with otorrhea. If untreated, it can develop into chronic suppurative otitis media (see the section on chronic suppurative otitis media in Chapter 8, "Complications and Sequelae"). Several clinical trials have demonstrated that ototopical agents, such as ofloxacin otic solution 0.3% (Floxin Otic) and ciprofloxacin-dexamethasone (CiproDex), are effective when acute otorrhea occurs through a tympanostomy tube, even in the absence of a systemic anti-microbial agent (Dohar et al, 1996, 1999; Goldblatt et al, 1998; Roland, 2001). CiproDex has been shown to be more

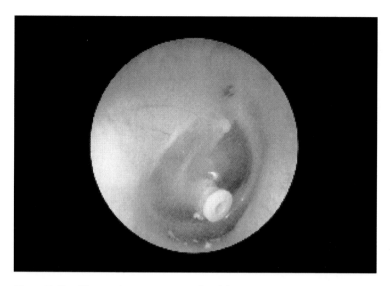

Figure 7–5 Otoscopic appearance of a right tympanic membrane with a grommet tympanostomy tube in place. Note the appearance of tiny white plaques around the tube (myringosclerosis), which is "cosmetic" and does not affect hearing. Reproduced from Bluestone CD. Conquering otitis media. Hamilton (ON): BC Decker; 1999.

effective than Floxin Otic. The use of other ototopical agents has not been approved by the US Food and Drug Administration (FDA), and they can be ototoxic when the tympanic membrane is not intact, especially ones that contain an aminoglycoside, such as neomycin, polymyxin B sulfate, and hydrocortisone otic suspension (Pediotic Suspension).

Adenoidectomy, in conjunction with myringotomy with and without tympanostomy tube placement, has been shown to be effective for chronic effusions in two large well-controlled clinical trials in children (Gates et al, 1987; Paradise et al, 1990). Our preference is to recommend only tympanostomy tube insertion if the child has not had them inserted in the past and does not have nasal obstruction caused by adenoid hypertrophy. This is because our studies (Mandel et al, 1989, 1992) showed that about half of the subjects did not require another operation. If obstructive adenoids are present, we recommend their removal at the initial procedure. For those children who have recurrence of chronic effusion following extrusion of the tubes and need a second surgical procedure, we advise an adenoidectomy, irrespective of adenoid size, with myringotomy. The decision to place tympanostomy tubes at this operation is on an individualized basis. Although the official government guideline recommended against adenoidectomy—in the absence of adenoid pathology—for this indication in children under the age of 4 years (Stool et al, 1994), our Pittsburgh trial showed that the procedure was also effective for subjects in this age group (Paradise et al, 1990). This difference of opinion has been discussed in detail elsewhere (Bluestone and Klein, 1995).

Tonsillectomy in conjunction with adenoidectomy for chronic effusions has been shown in a clinical trial in Great Britain to provide no significant benefit over adenoidectomy alone (Maw, 1983), and we do not recommend their removal unless there are other compelling indications, such as frequently recurrent throat infections (Paradise et al, 1984) or severe airway obstruction secondary to grossly enlarged tonsils.

CONCLUSION

Currently, management of patients with otitis media is going through a period of re-evaluation owing to several factors, including the steadily increasing incidence of the disease, which has been attributed to the ever-increasing rise in attendance in child day care, the dramatic emergence of multidrug-resistant bacterial pathogens, and the growing financial impact in today's cost-conscious climate. However, we now have enough information that is evidence based to either actively treat or not treat (observe) this disease. Using this information, we can now provide a more rational management plan, which, it is hoped, will stem the rise of antibiotic-resistant bacteria and be more cost effective, while still providing our patients with optimum health care.

REFERENCES

Barnett ED, Teele DW, Klein JO, et al. Comparison of ceftriaxone and trimethoprim-sulfamethoxazole for acute otitis media. Greater Boston Otitis Media Study Group. Pediatrics 1997;99:23–8.

Berman S, Byrns PJ, Bondy J, et al. Otitis media-related antibiotic prescribing patterns, outcomes and expenditures in a pediatric Medicaid population. Pediatrics 1997;100:585–92.

Bluestone CD. Pneumococcal conjugate vaccine: impact on otitis media and otolaryngology. Arch Otolaryngol Head Neck Surg 2001;127:464–7.

Bluestone CD, Klein JO. Clinical practice guideline on otitis media with effusion in young children: strengths and weaknesses. Otolaryngol Head Neck Surg 1995;112:507–11.

Bluestone CD, Klein JO, Gates GA. "Appropriateness" of tympanostomy tubes. Setting the record straight. Arch Otolaryngol Head Neck Surg 1994;120:1051–3.

Cantekin EI, Mandel EM, Bluestone CD, et al. Lack of efficacy of a decongestant-antihistamine combination for otitis media with effusion ("secretory" otitis media) in children. N Engl J Med 1983;308:297–301.

Casselbrant ML, Brostoff LM, Cantekin EI, et al. Otitis media with effusion in preschool children. Laryngoscope 1985;95:428–36.

Casselbrant ML, Kaleida PH, Rockette HE, et al. Efficacy of antimicrobial prophylaxis and of tympanostomy tube insertion for prevention of recurrent acute otitis media: results of a randomized clinical trial. Pediatr Infect Dis J 1992;11:278–86.

Chan KH, Bluestone CD. Lack of efficacy of middle-ear inflation: treatment of otitis media with effusion in children. Otolaryngol Head Neck Surg 1989;100:317–23.

Culpepper L, Froom J. Routine antimicrobial treatment of acute otitis media: is it necessary? JAMA 1997;278:1643–5.

Dohar JE, Alper CM, Bluestone CD, et al. Treatment of chronic suppurative otitis media with topical ciprofloxacin. In: Lim DJ, Bluestone CD, Casselbrant ML, et al, editors. Recent advances in otitis media: proceedings of the Sixth International Symposium. Hamilton (ON): BC Decker; 1996. p. 525–8.

Dohar JE, Garner ET, Nielsen RW, et al. Topical ofloxacin treatment of otorrhea in children with tympanostomy tubes. Arch Otolaryngol Head Neck Surg 1999;125:537–45.

Dowell SF, Marcy SM, Phillips WR, et al. Otitis media—principles of judicious use of antimicrobial agents. In: Dowell SF, editor. Principles of judicious use of antimicrobial agents for pediatric upper respiratory tract infections. Pediatrics 1998;101 Suppl:165–6.

Fireman B, Black SB, Shinefield HR, et al. Impact of the pneumococcal conjugate vaccine on otitis media. Pediatr Infect Dis J 2003;22: 10–6.

Fria TJ, Cantekin EI, Eichler JA. Hearing acuity of children with otitis media with effusion. Arch Otolaryngol Head Neck Surg 1985;111: 10–6.

Gates FA, Avery CA, Prihoda TJ, Cooper JJ Jr. Effectiveness of adenoidectomy and tympanostomy tubes in the treatment of chronic otitis media with effusion. N Engl J Med 1987;317:1444–51.

Goldblatt EL, Dohar J, Nozza RJ et al. Topical ofloxacin versus systemic amoxicillin/clavulanate in purulent otorrhea in children with tympanostomy tubes. Int J Pediatr Otorhinolaryngol 1998;46:91–6.

Hendley JO. Clinical practice. Otitis media. N Engl J Med 2002;347: 1169–74.

Howie VM, Ploussard JH. Efficacy of fixed combination antibiotics versus separate components in otitis media. Clin Pediatr 1972;11: 205–14.

Hyde TB, Gay K, Stephens DS, et al. Macrolide resistance among invasive *Streptococcus pneumoniae* isolates. JAMA 2001;286:1857–62.

Kaleida PH, Bluestone CD, Rockette HE, et al. Amoxicillin-clavulanate potassium compared with cefaclor for acute otitis media in infants and children. Pediatr Infect Dis J 1987;6:265–71.

Kaleida PH, Casselbrant ML, Rockette HE, et al. Amoxicillin or myringotomy or both for acute otitis media: results of a randomized clinical trial. Pediatrics 1991;87:466–74.

Kay DJ, Nelson M, Rosenfeld RM. Meta-analysis of tympanostomy tube sequelae. Otolaryngol Head Neck Surg 2001;124:374–80.

Lahikainen EA. Clinico-bacteriologic studies on acute otitis media: aspiration of tympanum as diagnostic and therapeutic method. Acta Otolaryngol (Stockh) 1953;107:1.

Mandel EM, Casselbrant ML, Kurs-Lasky M, Bluestone CD. Efficacy of ceftibuten compared with amoxicillin for otitis media with effusion in infants and children. Pediatr Infect Dis J 1996;14:281–91.

Mandel EM, Casselbrant ML, Rockette HE, Bluestone CD. Efficacy of 20- vs. 10-day antimicrobial treatment for acute otitis media. Pediatrics 1995;96:5–13.

Mandel EM, Casselbrant ML, Rockette HE, et al. Systemic steroid for chronic otitis media with effusion in children. Pediatrics 2002;110: 1071–80.

Mandel EM, Kardatzke D, Bluestone CD, Rockette HE. A comparative evaluation of cefaclor and amoxicillin in the treatment of acute otitis media. Pediatr Infect Dis J 1993;12:726–32.

Mandel EM, Rockette HE, Bluestone CD, et al. Efficacy of amoxicillin with and without decongestant-antihistamine for otitis media with effusion in children. N Engl J Med 1987;316:432–7.

Mandel EM, Rockette HE, Bluestone CD, et al. Myringotomy with and without tympanostomy tubes for chronic otitis media with effusion. Arch Otolaryngol Head Neck Surg 1989;115:1217–24.

Mandel EM, Rockette HE, Bluestone CD, et al. Efficacy of myringotomy with and without tympanostomy tubes for chronic otitis media with effusion. Pediatr Infect Dis J 1992;11:270–7.

Mandel EM, Rockette HE, Paradise JL, et al. Comparative efficacy of erythromycin-sulfisoxazole, cefaclor, amoxicillin or placebo for otitis media with effusion in children. Pediatr Infect Dis J 1991;10: 899–906.

Maw AR. Chronic otitis media with effusion and adenotonsillectomy. A prospective randomized controlled study. BMJ 1983;87:1586–8.

Paradise JL. Short-course antimicrobial treatment for acute otitis media: not best for infants and young children. JAMA 1997;278:1640–2.

Paradise JL, Bluestone CD, Bachman RZ, et al. Efficacy of tonsillectomy for recurrent throat infection in severely affected children. Results of parallel randomized and nonrandomized clinical trials. N Engl J Med 1984;310:674–83.

Paradise JL, Bluestone CD, Colborn DK, et al. Adenoidectomy and adenotonsillectomy for recurrent acute otitis media: parallel randomized clinical trials in children not previously treated with tympanostomy tubes. JAMA 1999;282:945–53.

Paradise JL, Bluestone CD, Rogers KD, et al. Efficacy of adenoidectomy for recurrent otitis media in children previously treated with tympanostomy-tube placement: results of parallel randomized and nonrandomized trials. JAMA 1990;263:2066–73.

Paradise JL, Haggard MP, Lous J, et al. Developmental implications of early-life otitis media. Int J Pediatr Otorhinolaryngol 1995;32: S37–44.

Pelton SI, Klein JO. The future of pneumococcal conjugate vaccines for prevention of pneumococcal diseases in infants and children. Pediatrics 2002;110:805–14.

Roland PS. Topical dexamethasone enhances resolution of acute otitis media with a tympanostomy tube [abstract]. In: Combined otolaryngological spring meetings of the Triological Society and the American Society of Pediatric Otolaryngology; 2001 May 14; Boca Raton, FL.

Rosenfeld RM, Bluestone CD. Evidence-based otitis media. Hamilton (ON): BC Decker; 1999.

Rosenfeld RM, Mandel EM, Bluestone CD. Systemic steroids for otitis media with effusion in children. Arch Otolaryngol Head Neck Surg 1991;117:984–9.

Rosenfeld RM, Post JC. Meta-analysis of antibiotics for the treatment of otitis media with effusion. Otolaryngol Head Neck Surg 1992; 106:378–86.

Rosenfeld RM, Vertrees JE, Carr J, et al. Clinical efficacy of antimicrobial drugs for acute otitis media: metaanalysis of 5400 children from thirty-three randomized trials. J Pediatr 1994;124:355–67.

Rudberg RD. Acute otitis media: comparative therapeutic results of sulfonamide and penicillin administered in various forms. Acta Otolaryngol (Stockh) 1954;113:1–79.

Schrag SJ, Pena C, Fernandez J, et al. Effect of short-course, high-dose amoxicillin therapy on resistant pneumococcal carriage. A randomized trial. JAMA 2001;286:49–56.

Stool SE, Berg AO, Berman S, et al. Otitis media with effusion in young children. Clinical practice guideline, number 1 2. Rockville (MD): Agency for Health Care Policy and Research, Public Health Service, US Department of Health and Human Services; July 1994. AHCPR Publication No.: 94-0622.

Teele DW, Klein JO, Rosner B, et al. Epidemiology of otitis media during the first seven years of life in children in Greater Boston: a prospective, cohort study. J Infect Dis 1989;160:83–9.

Teele DW, Klein JO, Rosner B, et al. Middle ear disease and the practice of pediatrics. Burden during the first five years of life. JAMA 1983; 249:1026–9.

van Balen FA, de Melker RA, Touw-Otten FW. Double-blind randomized trial of co-amoxiclav versus placebo for persistent otitis media with effusion in Faeral practice. Lancet 1996;348:713–6.

van Buchem FL, Dunk JH, van't Hof MA. Therapy of acute otitis media: myringotomy, antibiotics or neither? A double-blind study in children. Lancet 1981;ii:883–7.

Williams RL, Chalmers TC, Stange KC, et al. Use of antibiotics in preventing recurrent acute otitis media and in treating otitis media with effusion. JAMA 1993;270:1344–51.

CHAPTER 8

COMPLICATIONS AND SEQUELAE

Complications from a middle ear infection still occur in the era of antibiotics because the middle ear is connected to the mastoid cells and adjacent to the inner ear and intracranial cavity. Complications in these regions are the most serious suppurative complications (Figure 8-1).

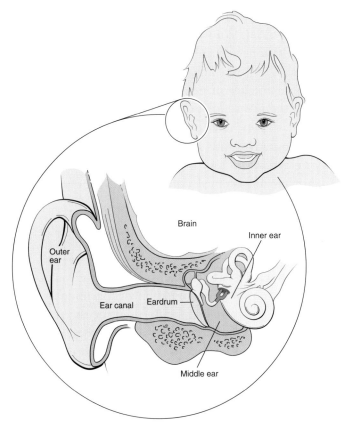

Figure 8–1 Middle ear infections can spread to adjacent structures such as the inner ear and brain. Reproduced from Bluestone CD. Conquering otitis media. Hamilton (ON): BC Decker; 1999.

Specific signs and symptoms are associated with otitis media and its complications and sequelae that should alert the clinician that one or more of them are present. Table 8-1 lists these signs and symptoms. Some of these diseases or disorders may be both a complication and a sequela, such as hearing loss. Another disease or disorder that is concurrent with the otitis media is considered a *complication*, whereas a *sequela* of otitis media is a disease or disorder that follows, is a consequence of, or is caused by otitis media.

For most of these complications and sequelae, the primary care clinician should consult with an otolaryngologist, and, for some, consultation with an expert in infectious disease is also appropriate. When an intracranial suppurative complication develops, a neurologist or neurosurgeon will also be an important part of the management team.

One of the most common and troubling sequelae is chronic suppurative otitis media. If not promptly and appropriately treated, it can lead to other complications and sequelae, such as an intracranial complication, which can be life threatening.

CHRONIC SUPPURATIVE OTITIS MEDIA

Chronic suppurative otitis media is the stage of ear disease in which there is chronic inflammation of the middle ear cleft (*middle ear cleft* is a term frequently used for the middle ear, eustachian tube, and mastoid gas cells) and chronic perforation of the tympanic membrane. Mastoiditis is invariably a part of the pathologic process. Otorrhea is almost always present. There is no consensus regarding the duration of otitis media to be designated *chronic suppurative otitis media*, but it can be even as short as 3 weeks, especially when the causative organism is *Pseudomonas*. Chronic suppurative otitis media is a major

Table 8–1 Signs and Symptoms Associated with a Complication or Sequela of Otitis Media

Intratemporal (Extracranial)
Otalgia (severe)
Otorrhea (profuse)
Hearing loss (moderate to severe conductive or sensorineural of any degree)
Vertigo
Nystagmus
Postauricular erythema/swelling/pain/tenderness
Protrusion of pinna
Facial paralysis

Intracranial
Presumptive
Headache (persistent/moderate to severe)
Lethargy
Malaise
Irritability
Otalgia (severe)
Fever (high/onset during episode of otitis media)
Nausea (moderate to severe)
Vomiting
Definitive
Neck stiffness
Focal seizures
Ataxia
Blurred vision
Papilledema
Diplopia
Hemiplegia
Aphasia
Dysdiadochokinesia
Intension tremor
Dysmetria
Hemianopia

health problem in many populations around the world, affecting diverse racial and cultural groups living not only in temperate climates but also in climate extremes ranging from the Arctic Circle to the equator (Bluestone, 1998b).

The etiology and pathogenesis of chronic suppurative otitis media are multifactorial, but they usually begin with an episode of acute otitis media. Thus, the factors that have been associated with acute otitis media may be initially involved, such as an upper respiratory tract infection, anatomic factors such as eustachian tube dysfunction, host factors such as young age, immature or impaired immunologic status, presence of an upper respiratory allergy, familial predisposition, presence of older siblings in the household, male sex, race, method of feeding (bottle versus breast), and environmental (eg, smoking in the household) and social factors. Probably the most important factors related to the onset of acute otitis media in infants and young children are immaturity of the structure and function of the eustachian tube and immaturity of the immune system (Bluestone, 1996).

Acute otitis media with perforation (or when a tympanostomy tube is present) usually *precedes* chronic suppurative otitis media. Because a spontaneous perforation commonly accompanies an episode of acute otitis media that is untreated with an antimicrobial agent, and less commonly despite adequate treatment, it may be part of the natural history of the disease process rather than a complication. But it is important to note that chronic ear infection is preceded by an acute ear infection.

When a chronic perforation or tympanostomy tube is present and there is no evidence of infection, reinfection probably occurs in one of two ways. Bacteria from the nasopharynx gain access to the middle ear owing to *reflux* or *insufflation* of nasopharyngeal secretions (owing to crying in the infant, nose blowing, or swallowing when there is nasal obstruction present, ie, the "Toynbee phenomenon" [Bluestone et al,

1974]) through the eustachian tube because the middle ear *air cushion* is lost; an episode usually occurs with an upper respiratory tract infection (see Figure 4-10 in Chapter 4, "Pathogenesis"). In most instances, these bacteria are initially the same as those isolated when acute otitis media occurs behind an intact tympanic membrane, such as *Streptococcus pneumoniae* and *Haemophilus influenzae* (Mandel et al, 1994). Following the acute otorrhea, *Pseudomonas aeruginosa*, *Staphylococcus aureus*, and other organisms from the external ear canal enter the middle ear through the nonintact tympanic membrane, which results in *secondary* infection and acute otorrhea and chronic suppurative otitis media. The second way it can occur is when the middle ear cleft is contaminated by organisms (eg, *P. aeruginosa*, *S. aureus*) present in water that enters the nonintact eardrum during bathing and swimming (Bluestone, 1998a).

As stated above, the bacteria that cause the initial episode of acute otitis media and perforation or acute otorrhea through a tympanostomy tube are usually not those that are isolated from chronic suppurative otitis media (Mandel et al, 1994). The most common organism isolated from around the world when chronic otitis media is the diagnosis is *P. aeruginosa*. *S. aureus* is also found, but less commonly (Indudharan et al, 1999; Kenna et al, 1986). Table 8-2 shows that frequency of bacteria isolated from children with chronic suppurative otitis media at the Children's Hospital of Pittsburgh (Kenna et al, 1993). Anaerobic bacteria were isolated infrequently in this study. The diagnosis of chronic suppurative otitis media is usually evident from the otoscopic examination (Figure 8-2).

Chronic purulent, mucoid, or serous discharge through a perforation of the tympanic membrane is evidence of chronic suppurative otitis media. Frequently, a polyp will be seen emerging through the perforation or tympanostomy tube. There is no otalgia, mastoid or pinna tenderness, vertigo, or fever. When any of these signs or symptoms are present, the

Table 8–2 Bacteriology of Otorrhea in 51 Children (80 Ears) with Chronic Suppurative Otitis Media

Bacteria Isolated	Number of Isolates* ($n = 118$)
Pseudomonas aeruginosa	56
Staphylococcus aureus	18
Diphtheroids	8
Streptococcus pneumoniae	7
Haemophilus influenzae (nontypeable)	6
Bacteroides sp	2
Candida parapsilosis	2
Enterococcus	2
Acinetobacter	2
Staphylococcus epidermidis	1
Morganella morgagni	1
Providencia stuartii	1
Klebsiella sp	1
Proteus sp	1
Serratia marcescens	1
Moraxella	1
Pseudomonas cepacia	1
Providencia rettgeri	1
Pseudomonas maltophilia	1
Achromobacter xylosoxidans	1
Eikenella	1

*Number exceeds 80 because of more than one organism isolated in 38 ears.
Adapted from Kenna et al, 1993.

examiner should look for a possible suppurative intratemporal complication, such as mastoiditis or labyrinthitis, or an intracranial complication (discussed later in this chapter). A search for the underlying cause of the infection may reveal the presence of paranasal sinusitis, which must be actively treated because the ear infection may not respond to medical treatment until the sinusitis resolves. An upper respiratory tract allergy or a nasopharyngeal tumor may also contribute to the pathogenesis of chronic suppurative otitis media and will need to be managed appropriately. The discharge should be appro-

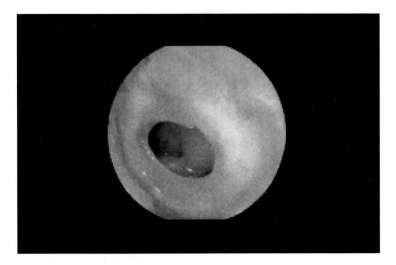

Figure 8–2 Otoscopic appearance of perforated tympanic membrane in which there has been chronic otorrhea. Reproduced from Bluestone CD. Conquering otitis media. Hamilton (ON): BC Decker; 1999.

priately examined by a Gram-stained smear and cultured for causative organisms, and susceptibility studies should also be obtained. One of the most important parts of the evaluation is a complete examination of the ear canal, tympanic membrane, and, if the perforation is large enough, the middle ear. This should be done with the aid of the otomicroscope. A search for a polyp or unsuspected cholesteatoma or neoplasm should also be conducted. Computed tomographic (CT) scans of the middle ear and mastoid should be obtained when intensive medical treatment (including intravenous antimicrobial therapy) fails.

Treatment of chronic suppurative otitis media is initially medical and directed toward eliminating the infection from the middle ear and mastoid. Because bacteria most frequently cultured are gram negative, antimicrobial agents should be selected to be effective against these organisms. Some experts currently advocate the use ototopical agents as first-line treatment (Hannley et al, 2000).

OTOTOPICAL MEDICATIONS

A suspension containing polymyxin B, neomycin sulfates, and hydrocortisone (Pediotic), one that has neomycin, polymyxin E, and hydrocortisone (Coly-Mycin), has been used in the past. Caution is advised owing to the concern over the potential ototoxicity of these agents (Perry and Smith, 1996; Podoshin et al, 1989; Roland, 1994; Welling et al, 1995). In addition, a recent in vitro susceptibility study showed that only 18% of middle ear isolates were sensitive to topical neomycin (Dohar et al, 1996a). Some clinicians use topical tobramycin (with dexamethasone) (Tobradex) or gentamicin (Garamycin) ophthalmic drops instilled into the ear when *Pseudomonas* is isolated, but, again, these agents are aminoglycosides and may therefore be ototoxic (Browning et al, 1988; Brummett et al, 1976; Gyde, 1976; Ikeda and Morizono, 1991; Meyerhoff et al, 1983). More importantly, none of these popular medications are approved for use when there is a nonintact tympanic membrane.

The US Food and Drug Administration has approved ofloxacin (Floxin Otic), an ototopical agent, for use in children when acute otitis media with otorrhea occurs when a tympanostomy tube is in place. It has been demonstrated to be safe and effective (Dohar et al, 1999; Goldblatt et al, 1998) and approved for this indication in children. It is also approved for adults who have chronic suppurative otitis media, but it is currently not approved for this indication in children (Agro et al, 1998), even though it has been reported to be effective in this age group (Kaga and Ichimura, 1998). Topical ofloxacin has been shown to be more effective than the combination of neomycin-polymyxin B-hydrocortisone otic drops in adults with chronic suppurative otitis media (Tong et al, 1996).

Ciprofloxacin with dexamethasone (CiproDex) has recently been approved to treat acute otitis media when a tympanostomy tube is in the tympanic membrane and has been shown to be more effective than Floxin Otic for this indication. Even though ciprofloxacin is not approved for chronic suppurative otitis media, it appears to be effective (Aslan et al, 1998; Dohar et al, 1996b; Esposito et al, 1990, 1992). One study showed that topical ciprofloxacin was more effective than topical gentamicin for chronic suppurative otitis media in adults (Tutkun et al, 1995), and another showed that this antibiotic was equally effective as tobramycin in adults with this infection (Fradis et al, 1997). No apparent ototoxicity occurred after using this ototopical agent in patients with chronic suppurative otitis media (Ozagar et al, 1997). In addition, topical ciprofloxacin did not cause ototoxicity in the monkey model of chronic suppurative otitis media (Alper et al, 1999). There is still no consensus about the potential efficacy of adding a corticosteroid component to the antimicrobial agent, but corticosteroids may hasten resolution of the inflammation (Crowther and Simpson, 1991). Recently, Alper and associates (2000) reported that the combination of tobramycin and dexamethasone was more effective than tobramycin alone in the monkey model of chronic suppurative otitis media. Tobramycin with and without dexamethasone was not only effective but also safe, that is, there was no cochlear damage.

Thus, the lack of reported clinical trials in children notwithstanding, it seems reasonable today to use CiproDex (and Floxin Otic as an alternative) initially in children who have uncomplicated chronic suppurative otitis media.

As an alternative to an antibiotic topical agent, some clinicians recommend antiseptic drops. An antiseptic ototopical agent (aluminum acetate) was found to be as effective as topical gentamicin sulfate for otorrhea in a randomized clinical trial reported from the United Kingdom (Clayton et al, 1990). Thorp and colleagues (1998) evaluated the in vitro activity of acetic acid and aluminum subacetate (Burow's solution) and found both to be effective against the major pathogens causing chronic suppurative otitis media. Burow's solution was somewhat more effective than acetic acid. Antiseptic drops (eg, acetic acid) are commonly used in underdeveloped countries and are reputed to be effective. Owing to cost and availability, antibiotic ototopical agents are used when antiseptic drops are ineffective.

SYSTEMIC ANTIMICROBIAL THERAPY

Systemic oral antimicrobial agents may be used if the bacterium is susceptible to the currently approved drugs. There is still a restriction in using the quinolones in children under the age of 17 years, which remains a problem today because the most common bacterial pathogen is *Pseudomonas*. However, these agents can be effective. If the patient is a treatment failure following the administration of ototopical agents, with or without an oral antimicrobial agent, the patient should receive a parenteral β-lactam antipseudomonal drug, such as ticarcillin, piperacillin, or ceftazidime. Empirically, ticarcillin-clavulanate is usually selected because *Pseudomonas*, with and without *S. aureus*, is frequently isolated. The results of the culture and susceptibility studies dictate the antimicrobial agent ultimately chosen (Kenna et al, 1986, 1993). Dagan and colleagues (1992) in Israel and Arguedas and associates (1993) in Costa Rica reported excellent results using ceftazidime. In Finland, Vartiainen and Kansanen (1992) also recommend a trial of intravenous antimicrobial therapy before considering mastoid surgery. The regimen can be altered when the results of culture and susceptibility tests are available. Also, the external canal purulent material and debris (and middle ear, if possible) are aspirated and the ototopical medication is instilled daily. This method of treatment can be administered with the child hospitalized but is more cost-effective and probably just as effective on an ambulatory basis (Dagan et al, 1992; Esposito, 2000).

In about 90% of children, the middle ear will be free of discharge and the signs of chronic suppurative otitis media will be greatly improved or absent within 5 to 7 days. Kenna and colleagues (1986) conducted a study in 36 pediatric patients with chronic suppurative otitis media in which all received parenteral antimicrobial therapy and daily aural toilet. Medical therapy alone resolved the infection in 32 patients (89%); 4 children required tympanomastoidectomy. The investigators later increased the study group to 66 children and reported similar short-term results; 89% had *dry* ears following intravenous antibiotic therapy (Kenna and Bluestone, 1988). In a follow-up of that study, 51 of the original 66 were evaluated for their long-term outcomes (Kenna et al, 1993). Of these 51 children, 40 (78%) had resolution of their initial or recurrent infection following medical treatment and 11 (22%) had to eventually have mastoid surgery. Failure was associated with older children and an early recurrence. Englender and colleagues (1990) did serotyping and pyocin typing of *P. aeruginosa* of 142 patients, including children, and found that if the patient had a recurrence with a different type, medical treatment was frequently successful. If the patient had recurrence of the otorrhea with the same type, medical therapy usually failed, and the patient required mastoid surgery. Leiberman and coworkers (1992) found that when children had an early recurrence, they were less likely to benefit from either medical treatment, including intravenous antibiotics, or surgical management. (For details of the surgical technique of mastoidectomy for chronic suppurative otitis media, see Bluestone [2002].)

If resolution does not occur and hospitalization is not required, the child can be discharged and receive the parenteral antibiotic and ear drops (by the parent or caregiver) for a period of 10 to 14 days at home. The patient should be followed at periodic intervals to watch for signs of spontaneous closure of the perforation, which frequently happens after the middle ear and mastoid are no longer infected. Appropriate intensive medical treatment should be attempted before recommending major ear surgery because the outcome of surgery is not as favorable when medical treatment is withheld (Vartiainen and Vartiainen, 1996).

When chronic suppurative otitis media fails to respond to intensive medical therapy (ie, intravenous antibiotics, aural toilet, and ototopical medications) within several days, surgery on the middle ear and mastoid, that is, *tympanomastoidectomy*, may be required to eradicate the infection. A CT scan should be obtained (see earlier in this chapter). Failures usually occur when there is

- an underlying blockage of the communication between the middle ear and mastoid (ie, *aditus-ad-antrum*),
- irreversible chronic osteitis,
- cholesteatoma (or tumor), or
- an early recurrence with the same causative organism (Kenna et al, 1993).

PREVENTION OF RECURRENCE

With an understanding of the pathogenesis of chronic suppurative otitis media (ie, chronic otorrhea is preceded by acute otorrhea), the most effective way to prevent recurrence of otorrhea when the tympanic membrane is intact and an attack of acute otitis media occurs is to promptly, appropriately, and adequately treat the infection with the usual oral antimicrobial agents recommended for acute otitis media. If the tympanic membrane is not intact (ie, a perforation or a tympanostomy tube is present without evidence of infection), early treatment of acute otorrhea, that is, acute otitis media, should likewise be effective. Treatment with an oral antimicrobial agent may be enhanced by adding an ototopical agent(s) (eg, CiproDex) to prevent a secondary infection with external ear canal organisms, such as *Pseudomonas*.

When a perforation (or tympanostomy tube) is present but there is no middle ear–mastoid infection, and it is desirable to maintain middle ear ventilation through a nonintact eardrum, recurrent episodes of otorrhea can usually be prevented with *antimicrobial prophylaxis*, for example, amoxicillin (Maynard et al, 1972). If a tympanostomy tube is present and the middle ear is now disease free, its removal may restore middle ear–eustachian tube physiology (ie, prevent *reflux* or *insufflation* of nasopharyngeal secretions). Yet removal of tympanostomy tubes may not be desirable, especially in infants and young children. In these cases, antimicrobial prophylaxis should also be considered until the tubes spontaneously extrude.

If the child has a chronic perforation that is now dry, *tympanoplastic surgery* should be considered. The same factors should be considered when deciding to repair an eardrum perforation in children as described above related to removing a tympanostomy tube (Bluestone, 2002).

COMPLICATIONS AND SEQUELAE OTHER THAN CHRONIC SUPPURATIVE OTITIS MEDIA

The following are the complications and sequelae that occur within the intratemporal bone other than chronic suppurative otitis media.

Hearing Loss

Hearing loss is the most common complication and sequela of otitis media and can be *conductive, sensorineural,* or both. When conductive, the loss may be transient or permanent. When sensorineural in origin, the impairment is usually permanent.

Sensorineural hearing loss can be mild, moderate, severe, or profound. Reversible sensorineural hearing impairment is generally attributed to the effect of increased tension and stiffness of the round window membrane. Permanent sensorineural hearing loss is most likely attributable to the spread of infection or products of inflammation through the round window membrane into the labyrinth, development of a perilymphatic fistula in the oval or round window, or a suppurative complication such as labyrinthitis. This should prompt the primary care clinician to consult an otolaryngologist.

Vestibular, Balance, and Motor Dysfunctions

Otitis media is the most common cause of vestibular disturbance in children. Recent studies of labyrinthine function in children with and without middle ear effusion confirm that the vestibular system is adversely affected, and following tympanostomy tube placement, these dysfunctions return to normal (Casselbrant et al, 1995, 1998). Also, tests of motor proficiency have been demonstrated to be abnormal in children when middle ear effusion is present (Hart, 1998). In contrast to these dysfunctions related to middle ear effusion, the onset of vertigo associated with an episode of otitis media is usually indicative of labyrinthitis. This should signal referral to an otolaryngologist.

Perforation of the Tympanic Membrane

A perforation of the tympanic membrane can be acute or chronic, otitis media may or may not be present, and, when otitis media is present, otorrhea may or may not be present. Classification of perforation includes the site, extent, and duration of the perforation.

Acute perforation. One of the most common complications of acute otitis media is perforation of the tympanic membrane accompanied by acute otorrhea through the defect. This is known as *acute otitis media with perforation*. Also, an acute perforation can be present in which there is otitis media but no evidence of otorrhea. Acute otitis media with perforation was more frequently encountered before the widespread use of antimicrobial therapy, but it is still prevalent in developing countries, where primary health care is inadequate (Bluestone, 1998b).

When an attack of acute otitis media is complicated by a perforation (usually accompanied by otorrhea), one of four outcomes is possible: (1) resolution of the acute otitis media and healing of the tympanic membrane defect; (2) resolution of the acute otitis media, but the perforation becomes chronic; (3) the perforation and otitis media persist to become chronic, that is, *chronic suppurative otitis media* (see earlier in this chapter); or (4) a suppurative complication of otitis media develops (see later in this chapter).

Chronic perforation. Chronic perforation occurs when an acute perforation of the tympanic membrane fails to heal after 3 months or longer. A chronic perforation that is not associated with either acute otitis media or chronic suppurative otitis media frequently does not heal spontaneously and usually requires surgical repair, for example, myringoplasty or tympanoplasty. This is because the middle ear is susceptible to acute otitis media and subsequently to chronic suppurative otitis media when a perforation persists. This can result from contamination of the middle ear through the external auditory canal or by reflux of nasopharyngeal secretions into the middle ear (see Figure 4-11 in Chapter 4, "Pathogenesis").

Mastoiditis

Mastoiditis may or may not be a suppurative complication of otitis media because both acute otitis media and otitis media with effusion can also involve the mastoid. Mastoiditis may be acute, subacute, or chronic. The following is a classification of the stages of this suppurative complication that has recently been revised based on an understanding of the pathogenesis and pathology and on the more recent availability of CT scans (Bluestone, 1998a).

Acute mastoiditis.   Acute mastoiditis can be staged as follows: acute mastoiditis without periosteitis/osteitis, acute mastoiditis with periosteitis, and acute mastoid osteitis (with or without subperiosteal abscess).

Acute mastoiditis without periosteitis/osteitis is the natural extension and part of the pathologic process of acute middle ear infection. No periosteitis or osteitis of the mastoid is present. Most likely, all patients with acute otitis media probably have extension of the middle ear disease into the mastoid cell system, but this stage of acute mastoiditis is not strictly a complication of otitis media. It can nevertheless be misinterpreted as a complication of otitis media, especially when CT scans are obtained for other reasons during an episode of otitis media, for example, following head trauma. Specific signs or symptoms of mastoid infection such as protrusion of the pinna, postauricular swelling, tenderness, pain, or erythema are not present in this most common type of mastoiditis. This stage of mastoiditis can either resolve (most commonly with, or even without, treatment) or progress into a true complication of otitis media, that is, *acute mastoiditis with periosteitis*, which, in turn, can progress into *acute mastoid osteitis*.

Acute mastoiditis with periosteitis can develop when infection within the mastoid spreads to the periosteum covering the mastoid process. The route of infection from the mastoid cells to the periosteum is by venous channels, usually the mastoid emissary vein. This stage of acute mastoiditis should not be confused with the presence of a subperiosteal abscess. Acute mastoiditis with periosteitis is characterized by erythema, mild swelling, and tenderness in the postauricular area. The pinna may or may not be displaced inferiorly and anteriorly, with loss of the postauricular crease. Sagging of the posterior external auditory canal is infrequently present (Goldstein et al, 1998). Prompt antibiotic treatment is indicated, preferably culture directed following a tympanocentesis with myringotomy (see Chapter 6, "Diagnosis"). Even with appropriate management of this stage of mastoiditis, acute mastoid osteitis may develop.

Acute mastoid osteitis has also been termed *acute "coalescent" mastoiditis* or *acute surgical mastoiditis*, but the pathologic process is *osteitis*. When infection within the mastoid gas cell system progresses, rarefying osteitis can cause destruction of the bony trabeculae that separate the mastoid cells. The postauricular area is usually involved, but mastoid osteitis can occur without evidence of postauricular involvement. The signs and symptoms are similar to those described above for acute mastoiditis with periosteitis; a *subperiosteal abscess* may or may not be present (Figure 8-3). Management is similar to that described above when mastoiditis with periosteitis is present, but the addition of tympanostomy tube placement can enhance drainage for a longer period than myringotomy alone, and mastoidectomy is indicated.

There is a differential diagnosis between acute mastoiditis with cellulitis or osteitis and acute otitis externa with postauricular cellulitis. Acute mastoiditis with cellulitis or osteitis can be confused with acute otitis externa that has spread to the postauricular area. Both complications are characterized by protrusion of the pinna, postauricular swelling, erythema, and tenderness. Most commonly, these two complications can be

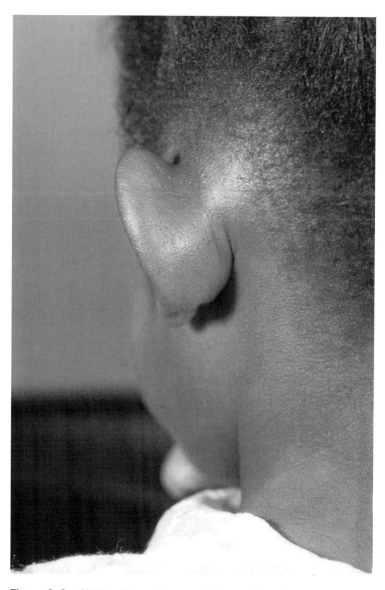

Figure 8–3 Child with acute mastoid osteitis with subperiosteal abscess. Reproduced from Bluestone CD. Conquering otitis media. Hamilton (ON): BC Decker; 1999.

distinguished by the condition of the postauricular crease. In acute mastoiditis, the crease is blunted or absent. When otitis externa is the diagnosis, the crease is usually present. Also, a history consistent with one or the other disease is helpful, and a complete examination of the external canal and pneumo-otoscopic evaluation of the tympanic membrane will frequently lead to the correct diagnosis (see Chapter 6, "Diagnosis"). Also, when there is an obvious postauricular subperiosteal abscess, the diagnosis is acute mastoiditis. However, both diseases can cause cervical lymphadenopathy. When the patient has severe pain and high fever and is seriously ill, and the diagnosis is uncertain between acute mastoiditis and acute otitis externa, a CT scan will usually distinguish between the two.

Subacute mastoiditis.   Subacute mastoiditis, although relatively uncommon, can develop if an acute middle ear and mastoid infection fails to totally resolve within the usual 10 to 14 days. This stage has also been termed *masked mastoiditis*. The classic signs and symptoms of acute mastoiditis such as pinna displacement, postauricular erythema, or subperiosteal abscess are usually absent, but otalgia with postauricular pain and fever may be present. The diagnosis is made by CT scan. In this stage, the infection in the mastoid can progress into another intratemporal complication or even an intracranial complication. Many cases of subacute mastoiditis occur in patients with persistent signs and symptoms of acute otitis media who, if initially administered antimicrobial treatment, are considered "treatment failures." When this condition occurs, tympanocentesis for diagnosis of the causative organism and myringotomy for drainage of the middle ear and mastoid in conjunction with culture-directed antimicrobial therapy will usually cure this condition without the need for mastoidectomy. If no middle ear effusion is present, the aditus ad antrum may be obstructed and the patient may require more aggressive management, such as mastoidectomy.

Chronic mastoiditis. Chronic mastoiditis is usually caused by *chronic suppurative otitis media* with a *chronic perforation* of the tympanic membrane. Chronic mastoiditis may also occur in the absence of chronic suppurative otitis media. Patients with relatively asymptomatic chronic otitis media with effusion frequently have some or all of the mastoid cell system involved in the chronic disease process. This is commonly visualized on CT scans of the temporal bones. Chronic infection may also be present in the mastoid, even in the absence of middle ear disease owing to obstruction of the aditus ad antrum; the otitis media resolved, but the disease in the mastoid did not. Symptoms can include low-grade fever and chronic otalgia and tenderness over the mastoid process. Management is described above (see earlier in this section under "Chronic Suppurative Otitis Media").

Petrositis

Infection from the middle ear and mastoid gas cells can spread into the petrosal gas cells of the mastoid apex, which is called *petrositis* or *petrous apicitis* or *apical petrositis*. This suppurative complication may be either acute or chronic and may result from acute otitis media or chronic ear disease. When chronic infection is the cause, it is usually attributable to chronic suppurative otitis media, cholesteatoma, or both. Consultation with an otolaryngologist is appropriate. The classic triad of signs and symptoms includes otitis media (usually with otorrhea), face pain, and cranial nerve IV palsy. The patient should be promptly referred to an otolaryngologist for management.

Labyrinthitis

When infection spreads from the middle ear, mastoid gas cells, or both into the cochlear and vestibular apparatus, the resulting complication is termed *labyrinthitis*. This complication can be either *serous labyrinthitis* (also termed *toxic labyrinthitis*) or *suppurative labyrinthitis*. Serous and suppurative labyrinthitis may be acute or chronic or circumscribed or generalized, respectively. The end stage of chronic labyrinthitis is termed *labyrinthine sclerosis*. The signs and symptoms are sensorineural hearing loss, vertigo, or both in association with an episode of acute otitis media. An otolaryngologist should be consulted promptly for appropriate management.

Facial Paralysis

Facial paralysis caused by otitis media or one of its complications or sequelae may be either acute or chronic (Figure 8-4). It may result from acute otitis media or chronic middle ear and mastoid disease, such as cholesteatoma, chronic suppurative otitis media, or both. An otolaryngologist should be consulted because management usually consists of tympanocentesis and myringotomy and tympanostomy tube placement when this complication occurs during an episode of acute otitis media. When chronic ear disease is present, the patient usually requires surgical intervention.

Otitis Externa

Acute otitis media with perforation and otorrhea or chronic suppurative otitis media can cause *otitis externa*. An infection in the mastoid may also erode the bone of the ear canal or the postauricular area, resulting in dermatitis. The skin of the ear canal is erythematous and edematous and is filled with purulent drainage, and yellow-crusted plaques may be present. The organisms involved are usually the same as those found in a middle ear–mastoid infection, but the flora of the external canal usually contribute to the infectious process. This complication is described in detail in the following section of this book ("Otitis Externa").

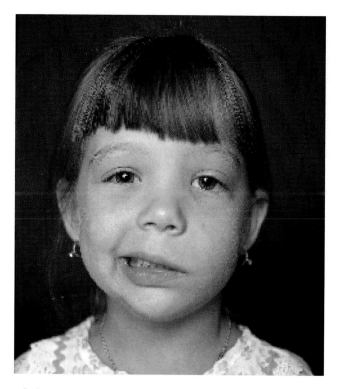

Figure 8–4 Facial paralysis in a child with acute otitis media. Reproduced from Bluestone CD. Conquering otitis media. Hamilton (ON): BC Decker; 1999.

Atelectasis of the Middle Ear–Tympanic Membrane and Retraction Pocket

Atelectasis of the middle ear is a sequela of eustachian tube dysfunction. Retraction or collapse of the tympanic membrane is characteristic of the condition; the tympanic membrane is a component of the lateral wall of the middle ear. Collapse implies passivity (absence of high negative middle ear pressure), whereas retraction implies active pulling inward of the tympanic membrane, usually from negative middle ear pressure, owing to eustachian tube dysfunction. Middle ear effusion is usually absent in atelectasis. The condition may be acute or chronic, localized (with or without a *retraction pocket*) or generalized, and mild, moderate, or severe (Figure 8-5). It is usually transient but can become chronic and may require placement of a tympanostomy tube to reverse the retraction pocket. It may even require tympanoplasty to prevent development of a cholesteatoma. Thus, referral to an otolaryngologist is appropriate when atelectasis is moderate to severe or if a retraction pocket persists.

Adhesive Otitis Media

Adhesive otitis media is a result of healing following chronic inflammation of the middle ear and mastoid. The mucous membrane is thickened by proliferation of fibrous tissue,

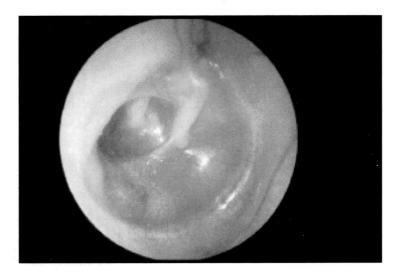

Figure 8–5 Retraction pocket in the posterosuperior quadrant of a right tympanic membrane. Reproduced from Bluestone CD. Conquering otitis media. Hamilton (ON): BC Decker; 1999.

which frequently impairs movement of the ossicles, resulting in conductive hearing loss. In addition to fixation of the ossicles, adhesive otitis media may be the cause of ossicular discontinuity and conductive hearing loss owing to rarefying ossicular osteitis, especially of the long process of the incus. Severe localized atelectasis (a retraction pocket) in the posterosuperior portion of the pars tensa of the tympanic membrane may cause adhesive changes to bind the tympanic membrane to the incus, stapes, and other surrounding middle ear structures and cause resorption of the ossicles. The development of a cholesteatoma then becomes possible.

Cholesteatoma

Cholesteatoma occurs when keratinizing stratified squamous epithelium accumulates in the middle ear or other pneumatized portions of the temporal bone. The term *aural* distinguishes this type of cholesteatoma from a similar pathologic entity that occurs outside the temporal bone. Cholesteatoma can be classified as *congenital* or *acquired*. The latter may be further subclassified as a sequela of otitis media (and certain related conditions) or as a result of implantation (iatrogenic or owing to trauma). Otitis media may also be involved in the pathogenesis of congenital cholesteatoma. Congenital cholesteatoma is not a sequela of otitis media, whereas acquired cholesteatoma is. Aural acquired cholesteatoma develops from a retraction pocket in the pars tensa or pars flaccida (see the earlier section in the chapter on atelectasis of the middle ear–tympanic membrane and retraction pocket), migration of epithelium through a preexisting defect of the tympanic membrane (eg, perforation) or, more rarely, metaplasia of the middle ear–mastoid mucous membrane. A cholesteatoma may involve only the middle ear, the mastoid, or both and may or may not extend beyond the temporal bone.

Classically, the diagnosis is made by the use of the otoscope to visualize a white mass in the tympanic membrane (Figure 8-6). Prompt referral to an otolaryngologist is indicated for surgical management.

Cholesterol Granuloma

Cholesterol granuloma is a relatively uncommon sequela of otitis media that is also called *idiopathic hemotympanum*. However, this term is a misnomer because there is no evidence of blood in the middle ear. The blue appearance of the tympanic membrane is most likely attributable to the reflection of light from the thick liquid (granuloma) within the middle ear. The tissue is composed of chronic granulations with foreign body giant cells, foam cells, and cholesterol crystals within the middle ear, the mastoid, or both. Surgical management is recommended.

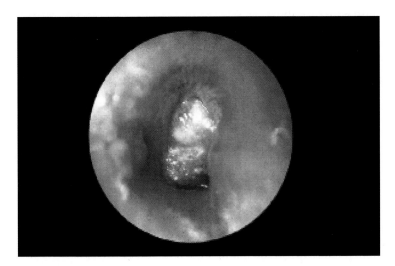

Figure 8–6 Otoscopic appearance of a cholesteatoma. Reproduced from Bluestone CD. Conquering otitis media. Hamilton (ON): BC Decker; 1999.

Tympanosclerosis

Tympanosclerosis is characterized by whitish plaques in the tympanic membrane and nodular deposits in the submucosal layers of the middle ear. The pathologic process occurs in the lamina propria in the tympanic membrane and affects the basement membrane if within the middle ear. Hyalinization is followed in both sites by deposition of calcium and phosphate crystals. Conductive hearing loss may occur if the ossicles become embedded in the deposits. Tympanosclerosis is usually a sequela of chronic middle ear disease (chronic otitis media with effusion or chronic suppurative otitis media) but is also associated with trauma, such as following tympanostomy tube insertion. Conductive hearing loss secondary to tympanosclerosis involving only the tympanic membrane is rare, although scarring of the eardrum at the site of tympanostomy tube insertion is common. Tympanosclerosis limited to the tympanic membrane and with little or no involvement of the middle ear and where the hearing is unaffected is common and is termed *myringosclerosis*. But extensive tympanosclerosis involving both the tympanic membrane and middle ear (involving the ossicles) will cause hearing loss. Management is difficult because recurrence is frequent after attempts at surgical correction.

Ossicular Discontinuity

Ossicular discontinuity, a sequela of otitis media and certain related conditions, is the result of rarefying osteitis caused by inflammation. A retraction pocket or cholesteatoma can also cause resorption of ossicles. The most commonly involved ossicle is the incus. Its long process usually erodes, resulting in a disarticulation of the incudostapedial joint. The second most commonly eroded ossicle is the stapes. Usually, the crural arches are initially involved. The malleus may also become eroded but not as commonly as the incus and stapes. Surgical repair (ossiculoplasty) is frequently successful in improving the hearing loss.

Ossicular Fixation

The ossicles can become fixed as a sequela of chronic middle ear inflammation, usually by fibrous tissue caused by adhesive otitis media, tympanosclerosis, or both. Each of these has a staging system for the extent and presence or absence of hearing loss. The ossicle itself or one or both of the joints (ie, incudostapedial or incudomalleolar) may be fixed. Surgical repair can frequently be successful in restoring hearing to normal or near-normal levels.

INTRACRANIAL COMPLICATIONS

There are seven intracranial suppurative complications of otitis media. These may be caused by an intratemporal complication such as mastoiditis, labyrinthitis, or one or more of the other complications of otitis media within the intracranial cavity (Figure 8-7). When any signs or symptoms (see Table 8-1) indicate one or more of these intracranial complications, prompt referral to an otolaryngologist, an infectious disease specialist, a neurologist, or a neurosurgeon is appropriate depending on the diagnosis. In addition, a history and complete physical examination (including a neurologic evaluation) and imaging of the temporal bones and intracranial cavity are critical in making the correct diagnosis.

Meningitis

Meningitis is an inflammation of the meninges that, when a suppurative complication of otitis media or certain related conditions such as labyrinthitis, is usually caused by a bac-

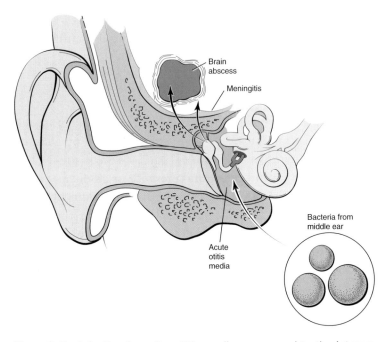

Figure 8–7 Infection from the otitis media can spread to the intracranial cavity, causing a suppurative complication. Reproduced from Bluestone CD. Conquering otitis media. Hamilton (ON): BC Decker; 1999.

terium associated with infections of the middle ear, the mastoid, or both. The infection may spread directly from the middle ear–mastoid through the dura and extend to the pia-arachnoid, causing generalized meningitis. Suppurative complications in an adjacent area, such as a subdural abscess, brain abscess, or lateral sinus thrombophlebitis, may also cause inflammation of the meninges.

Extradural Abscess

Extradural abscess, also termed *epidural abscess*, is an infection that occurs between the dura of the brain and the cranial bone. It usually results from the destruction of bone adjacent to the dura by cholesteatoma, chronic suppurative otitis media, or both. This occurs when granulation tissue and purulent material collect between the lateral aspect of the dura and the adjacent temporal bone. Dural granulation tissue within a bony defect is much more common than an actual accumulation of pus. When an abscess is present, a dural sinus thrombosis or, less commonly, a subdural or brain abscess may also be present.

Subdural Empyema

A *subdural empyema* occurs when purulent material collects within the potential space between the dura externally and the arachnoid membrane internally. Because the pus collects in a preformed space, it is correctly termed *empyema* rather than *abscess*. Subdural empyema may develop as a direct extension or, more rarely, by thrombophlebitis through venous channels.

Focal Otitic Encephalitis

Focal otitic encephalitis (also termed *cerebritis*) is a potential suppurative complication of acute otitis media, cholesteatoma, or chronic suppurative otitis media. It may also be a complication of one or more of the suppurative complications of these disorders, such as an extradural abscess or dural sinus thrombophlebitis, in which a focal area of the brain is edematous and inflamed. The signs and symptoms of this complication are similar to those associated with a brain abscess, but suppuration within the brain is not present.

Brain Abscess

Otogenic *brain abscess* is a potential intracranial suppurative complication of cholesteatoma, chronic suppurative otitis media, or both. It may also be caused by acute otitis media or acute mastoiditis. In addition, an intratemporal complication such as labyrinthitis or apical petrositis may be the focus, or the abscess may follow the development of an adjacent intracranial otogenic suppurative complication such as lateral sinus thrombophlebitis or meningitis.

Dural Sinus Thrombosis

Lateral and *sigmoid sinus thrombosis* or *thrombophlebitis* arises from inflammation in the adjacent mastoid. The superior and petrosal dural sinuses are also intimately associated with the temporal bone but are rarely affected. This suppurative complication can occur as a result of acute otitis media, an intratemporal complication (eg, acute mastoiditis or apical petrositis), or another intracranial complication of otitis media.

Otitic Hydrocephalus

Otitic hydrocephalus describes a complication of otitis media in which there is increased intracranial pressure without abnormalities of cerebrospinal fluid. The pathogenesis of the syndrome is unknown, but because the ventricles are not dilated, the term *benign intracranial hypertension* also seems appropriate. The disease is usually associated with lateral sinus thrombosis.

REFERENCES

Agro AS, Garner ET, Wright JW 3rd, et al. Clinical trial of ototopical ofloxacin for treatment of chronic suppurative otitis media. Clin Ther 1998;20:744–59.

Alper CM, Dohar JE, Gulhan M, et al. Treatment of chronic suppurative otitis media with topical tobramycin and dexamethasone. Arch Otolaryngol Head Neck Surg 2000;126:165–73.

Alper CM, Swarts, JD, Doyle WJ. Middle ear inflation for diagnosis and treatment of otitis media with effusion. Auris Nasus Larynx 1999; 26:479–86.

Arguedas AG, Herrera JF, Faingezicht I, et al. Ceftazidime for therapy of children with chronic suppurative otitis media without cholesteatoma. Pediatr Infect Dis J 1993;12:246–8.

Aslan A, Altuntas A, Titiz A, et al. A new dosage regimen for topical application of ciprofloxacin in the management of chronic suppurative otitis media. Otolaryngol Head Neck Surg 1998;118:883–5.

Bluestone CD. Pathogenesis of otitis media: role of the eustachian tube. Pediatr Infect Dis J 1996;14:281–91.

Bluestone CD. Acute and chronic mastoiditis and chronic suppurative otitis media. Semin Pediatr Infect Dis 1998a;9:12–26.

Bluestone CD. Epidemiology and pathogenesis of chronic suppurative otitis media: implications for prevention and treatment. Int J Pediatr Otorhinolaryngol 1998b;42:207–23.

Bluestone CD. Mastoiditis and cholesteatoma. In: Bluestone CD, Rosenfeld RS, editors. Surgical atlas of pediatric otolaryngology. Hamilton (ON): BC Decker; 2002:91–122.

Bluestone CD, Beery QC, Andrus S. Mechanics of the eustachian tube as it influences susceptibility to and persistence of middle-ear effusions in children. Ann Otol Rhinol Laryngol 1974;83:27–34.

Browning GG, Gatehouse S, Calder IT. Medical management of active chronic otitis media: a controlled study. J Laryngol Otol 1988;102:491–5.

Brummett RE, Harris RF, Lindgren JA. Detection of ototoxicity from drugs applied topically to the middle ear space. Laryngoscope 1976;86:1177–87.

Casselbrant ML, Furman JM, Rubenstein E, Mandel EM. Effect of otitis media on the vestibular system in children. Ann Otol Rhinol Laryngol 1995;104:620–4.

Casselbrant ML, Redfern MS, Furman JM, et al. Visual-induced postural sway in children with and without otitis media. Ann Otol Rhinol Laryngol 1998;107:401–5.

Clayton MI, Osborne JE, Rutherford D, Rivron RP. A double-blind, randomized, prospective trial of a topical antiseptic versus a topical antibiotic in the treatment of otorrhea. J Otolaryngol 1990;15:7–10.

Crowther JA, Simpson D. Medical treatment of chronic otitis media: steroid or antibiotic with steroid ear-drops? Clin Otolaryngol 1991;16:142–4.

Dagan R, Fliss DM, Einhorn M, et al. Outpatient management of chronic suppurative otitis media without cholesteatoma in children. Pediatr Infect Dis J 1992;11:542–6.

Dohar JE, Alper CM, Bluestone CD, et al. Treatment of chronic suppurative otitis media with topical ciprofloxacin. In: Lim, DJ, Bluestone CD, Casselbrant ML, et al, editors. Recent advances in otitis media: proceedings of the Sixth International Symposium. Hamilton (ON): BC Decker; 1996b. p. 525–8.

Dohar JE, Garner ET, Nielsen RW, et al. Topic ofloxacin treatment of otorrhea in children with tympanostomy tubes. Arch Otolaryngol Head Neck Surg 1999;125:537–45.

Dohar JE, Kenna MA, Wadowsky RM. In vitro susceptibility of aural isolates of *P. aeruginosa* to commonly used ototopical antibiotics. Am J Otol 1996a;17:207–9.

Englender M, Harell M, Guttman R, et al. Typing of *Pseudomonas aeruginosa* ear infections related to outcome of treatment. J Laryngol Otol 1990;104:678–81.

Esposito S. Outpatient parenteral treatment of bacterial infections: the Italian model as an international trend? J Antimicrob Chemother 2000;45:724–7.

Esposito S, D'Errico G, Montanaro C. Topical and oral treatment of chronic otitis media with ciprofloxacin. Arch Otolaryngol Head Neck Surg 1990;116:557–9.

Esposito S, Noviello S, D'Errico G, Montanaro C. Topical ciprofloxacin vs. intramuscular gentamicin for chronic otitis media. Arch Otolaryngol Head Neck Surg 1992;118:842–4.

Fradis M, Brodsky A, Ben-David J, et al. Chronic otitis media treated topically with ciprofloxacin or tobramycin. Arch Otolaryngol Head Neck Surg 1997;123:1057–60.

Goldblatt EL, Dohar J, Nozza RJ, et al. Topic ofloxacin versus systemic amoxicillin/clavulanate in purulent otorrhea in children with tympanostomy tubes. Int J Pediatr Otorhinolaryngol 1998;46:91–101.

Goldstein NA, Casselbrant ML, Bluestone CD, Kurs-Lasky M. Intratemporal complications of acute otitis media in infants and children. Otolaryngol Head Neck Surg 1998;119:444–54.

Gyde MC. When the weeping stopped: an otologist views otorrhea and gentamicin. Arch Otolaryngol 1976;102:542–6.

Hannley MT, Denneny JC, Holzer SS. Use of ototopical antibiotics in treating 3 common ear diseases. Otolaryngol Head Neck Surg 2000;122:934-40.

Hart MC. Childhood imbalance and chronic otitis media with effusion: effect of tympanostomy tube insertion on standardized tests of balance and locomotion. Laryngoscope 1998;108:665–70.

Ikeda K, Morizono T. Effect of ototopic application of a corticosteroid preparation on cochlear function. Am J Otolaryngol 1991;12: 150–3.

Indudharan R, Haq JA, Aiyar S. Antibiotics in chronic suppurative otitis media: a bacteriologic study. Ann Otol Rhinol Laryngol 1999; 108:440–5.

Kaga K, Ichimura K. A preliminary report: clinical effects of otic solution of ofloxacin in infantile myringitis and chronic otitis media. Int J Pediatr Otorhinolaryngol 1998;42:199–205.

Kenna MA, Bluestone CD. Medical management of chronic suppurative otitis media without cholesteatoma. In: Lim DJ, Bluestone CD, Klein JO, Nelson JD, editors. Recent advances in otitis media: proceedings of the Fourth International Symposium. Hamilton (ON): BC Decker; 1988. p. 222–6.

Kenna MA, Bluestone CD, Reilly J. Medical management of chronic suppurative otitis media without cholesteatoma in children. Laryngoscope 1986;96:146–51.

Kenna MA, Rosane BA, Bluestone CD. Medical management of chronic suppurative otitis media without cholesteatoma in children—update 1992. Am J Otolaryngol 1993;14:469–73.

Leiberman A, Fliss DM, Dagan R. Medical treatment of chronic suppurative otitis media without cholesteatoma in children— a two-year follow-up. Int J Pediatr Otorhinolaryngol 1992;24: 25–33.

Mandel EM, Casselbrant ML, Kurs-Lasky M. Acute otorrhea: bacteriology of a common complication of tympanostomy tubes. Ann Otol Rhinol Laryngol 1994;103:713–8.

Maynard JE, Fleshman JK, Tschopp CF. Otitis media in Alaskan Eskimo children: prospective evaluation of chemoprophylaxis. JAMA 1972; 219:597–9.

Meyerhoff WL, Morizono T, Shaddock LC, et al. Tympanostomy tubes and otic drops. Laryngoscope 1983;93:1022–7.

Ozagar A, Koc A, Ciprut A, et al. Effects of topical otic preparation on hearing in chronic otitis media. Otolaryngol Head Neck Surg 1997; 117:405–8.

Perry BP, Smith DW. Effect of Cortisporin Otic Suspension on cochlear function and efferent activity in the guinea pig. Laryngoscope 1996;106:1557–61.

Podoshin L, Fradis M, David B. Ototoxicity of ear drops in patients suffering from chronic otitis media. J Laryngol Otol 1989;103:46–50.

Roland PS. Clinical ototoxicity of topical antibiotic drops. Otolaryngol Head Neck Surg 1994;110:598–602.

Thorp MA, Kruger J, Oliver S, et al. The antibacterial acidity of acetic acid and Burow's solution as topical otological preparations. J Laryngol Otol 1998;112:925–8.

Tong MCF, Woo JKS, van Hasslet CA. A double-blind comparative study of ofloxacin otic drops versus neomycin-polymyxin B-hydrocortisone otic drops in the medical treatment of chronic suppurative otitis media. J Laryngol Otol 1996;110:309–14.

Tutkun A, Ozagar A, Koc A, et al. Treatment of chronic ear disease: topical ciprofloxacin vs. topical gentamicin. Arch Otolaryngol Head Neck Surg 1995;121:1414–6.

Vartiainen E, Kansanen M. Tympanomastoidectomy for chronic otitis media without cholesteatoma. Otolaryngol Head Neck Surg 1992; 106:230–4.

Vartiainen E, Vartiainen J. Effect of aerobic bacteriology on the clinical presentation and treatment results of chronic suppurative otitis media. J Laryngol Otol 1996;110:315–8.

Welling DB, Forrest LA, Goll F. Safety of ototopical antibiotics. Laryngoscope 1995;105:472–4.

CHAPTER 9

TERMINOLOGY, DEFINITIONS, AND CLASSIFICATION

Little has changed with respect to the terminology, classification, epidemiology, microbiology, and diagnostic modalities related to otitis externa. This is reassuring in an era of increased prevalence of resistant organisms underlying other infectious diseases of the ear, such as otitis media. Although all aspects of otitis externa are reviewed in the following chapters, the focus is on that aspect of disease management that has changed and likely will continue to change in the near future, namely, the newly developed ototopical agents.

Otitis externa is the generic term for any inflammatory condition of the external auditory meatus. It may be a local phenomenon or part of a generalized skin condition. Otitis externa may be acute, recurrent acute, or chronic. A classification of otitis externa is as follows:

Diffuse acute otitis externa is also known as "swimmer's ear."

Furunculosis is a focal infection of one of the hair follicles of the skin of the external auditory canal resulting from an obstructed apopilosebaceous gland and usually caused by *Staphylococcus aureus*.

Dermatitic otitis externa is dermatitis of the skin of the external auditory canal (eg, eczematoid, seborrheic, atopic, psoriatic).

Fungal otitis externa is otitis externa caused by a fungi.

Necrotizing ("malignant") otitis externa is skull base osteomyelitis.

In the United States, the incidence of otitis externa is cited as affecting 4 in 1,000 per year, of which 1% (4 in 100,000) go on to become chronic. This equates to over 5 million cases per year treated by American primary care physicians (Fields, 2002). Data collected from the 1998 National Ambulatory Medical Care Survey and The National Hospital Medical Care Survey for office, outpatient department, and emergency department visits revealed an estimate of 2,247,000 visits for International Classification of Diseases 9 codes 380.1 (otitis externa infective) and 380.2 (otitis externa other), or 0.22% of all visits (Ruben, 2001). An estimated 10% of all persons have suffered from "swimmer's ear" at some time in their lives (Raza, 1995).

REFERENCES

Fields M. Contin Med Educ J 2002;29:.

Raza SA, Denholm SW, Wong JC. An audit of the management of acute otitis externa in an ENT casualty clinic. J Laryngol Otol 1995;109; 130–3.

Ruben RJ. Efficacy of ofloxacin and other otic preparations for otitis externa. Pediatr Infect Dis 2001;20:108–10, 120–2.

CHAPTER 10

PHYSIOLOGY, EPIDEMIOLOGY, AND MICROBIOLOGY

To understand the pathophysiology of otitis externa, the normal anatomy and physiology of the external auditory canal must be understood. The external auditory canal is unique in being the only skin-lined cul-de-sac in the body, lined by a thin stratified squamous epithelium. Its lateral third is cartilaginous; the medial two-thirds are bony. The skin overlying the latter is thin and quite susceptible to trauma. Pathogens often gain access to the deeper layers of the epithelium as a result of minor abrasions or injuries to the skin lining the canal. It is one of the most pain-sensitive structures of the body.

The external auditory canal is warm and humid, and exfoliated skin provides an ideal growth medium for bacteria and fungi. The canal skin is unique in that it is continually migrating laterally, carrying debris with it. Cerumen is protective as it is acidic (pH 6.1–6.4) and hydrophobic, produced by pilosebaceous glands. In addition, it contains lysozymes that inhibit bacterial growth. Too much or too little cerumen predisposes to otitis externa. Hair helps prevent entry of foreign bodies. However, too much prevents migration and can predispose to cerumen impaction.

The normal external auditory canal should be self-cleaning. When it is not, there are a variety of ways of removing cerumen including irrigation, suction, mechanical removal, and ceruminolytics.

EPIDEMIOLOGY AND MICROBIOLOGY

Otitis externa occurs more frequently during the "swimming season." The cause is usually infective, although noninfectious and dermatologic processes should not be forgotten. Of the infectious causes, 80% are bacterial. The most common bacterial pathogens are *Pseudomonas aeruginosa* (most common), *Staphylococcus aureus*, and other gram-negative organisms such as *Enterococcus* species and *Proteus mirabilis* (Jones, 1997). These pathogens are in striking contrast to those that constitute the flora of the normal healthy external auditory canal, of which 96% are gram-positive organisms (*Staphylococcus epidermidis*, *Coryneform*, and streptococci-like species [Stroman et al, 2001]).

Before World War II, otitis externa was believed to be caused by fungal infection, and interest in studying the etiology of this disease was minimal. However, otitis externa entered the medical spotlight during the war because it was prevalent among American troops in the South Pacific. This disease became the second most common reason for lost duty among troops stationed in Guam (Gordon, 1948). Microbiologic studies initiated during World War II established that otitis externa is primarily bacterial in origin rather than fungal (Singer et al, 1952), which has been confirmed by subsequent studies (Agius et al, 1992; Hawke et al, 1984).

Fungi (and yeast) account for approximately 1% of the single isolates recovered from patients with acute otitis externa and are found in healthy ear canals in only 2.5%, with *Penicillium* being the most frequent genus identified (Roland and Stroman, 2002).

Curiously, *Candida albicans* was not found in healthy normal external auditory canals (Stroman et al, 2001). Fungi such as *Candida albicans* and *Aspergillus fumigatus*, when found, are generally considered pathogens, not saprophytes, given their distinct absence from healthy ear canals. Much has been said to the contrary, and it is critical to keep this in mind as few of the common ototopical therapies have antifungal spectrums of activity. Experience suggests that fungi may play a more important role in chronic infections and immunocompromised hosts. Although not confirmed, there is increasing concern that prolonged treatment with certain broad-spectrum ototopical antibiotics may also be a risk factor for development of fungal otitis externa.

Finally, viruses may also cause otitis externa. The most important cause of viral otitis externa is Ramsey Hunt syndrome, also called herpes zoster oticus. Total facial paralysis, hearing loss, and vertigo may result. Vesicular eruptions delineate a viral etiology from a bacterial or fungal one. Another important viral form of otitis externa is otitis externa hemorrhagica (bullous myringitis). Physical signs of hemorrhagic bulla on the tympanic membrane are pathognomonic.

REFERENCES

Agius AM, Pickles JM, Burch KL. A prospective study of otitis externa. Clin Otolaryngol 1992;17:150–4.

Gordon A. Otitis externa. Bull US Army Med Dept 1948;8:245–6.

Hawke M, Wong J, Krajden S. Clinical and microbiological features of otitis externa. J Otolaryngol 1984;13:289–95.

Jones RN, Milazzo J, Seidlin M. Ofloxacin otic solution for treatment of otitis externa in children and adults. Arch Otolaryngol Head Neck Surg 1997;123:1193–200.

Roland PS, Stroman DW. Microbiology of acute otitis externa. Laryngoscope 2002;112:1166–77.

Singer D, Freeman E, Hoffert E. Otitis externa: bacteriological and mycological studies. Ann Otol Rhinol Laryngol 1952;61:317–30.

Stroman DW, Roland PS, Dohar JE, Wayne B. Microbiology of healthy ears. Laryngoscope 2001;111:2054–9.

CHAPTER 11

PATHOGENESIS AND DIAGNOSIS

PATHOGENESIS

It has mistakenly been thought that water exposure causes otitis externa owing to bacterial contamination of the water infecting the external auditory canal on entry. This is now known to be untrue. The actual mechanism by which water entry leads to otitis externa is in altering the physiologic pH of the ear canal toward increased alkalinity, by removing other local protective factors, and by altering the normal homeostatic ecology.

There are some factors that can predispose individuals to otitis externa, including

- anatomic factors—a narrow canal, excessive wax production, hairy external auditory canal
- moisture—swimming, perspiration, high humidity
- high environmental temperatures
- mechanical removal of cerumen
- trauma—for example, insertion of cotton balls, fingernails, hearing aids, ear plugs, hair ornaments, and paper clips
- chronic dermatologic disease—for example, eczema, psoriasis, seborrheic dermatitis, and acne
- immunocompromise, including diabetes
- contaminated water (possible)

SYMPTOMS

The symptoms of otitis externa are distinct and generally helpful in distinguishing otitis externa from acute otitis media, the key entity in the differential diagnosis. Otitis externa symptoms include the following:

- pain and/or discomfort limited to the external auditory canal (itching through severe pain)

- deafness (conductive)
- pre- and postauricular lymph node enlargement/tenderness

SIGNS

The signs of otitis externa are diagnostic and include erythema and swelling of the external auditory canal skin with variable discharge or moist debris (Figure 11-1). More specific signs, such as periauricular vesicles, hyphae, bulla on the tympanic membrane, or granulation tissue, further distinguish the type of otitis externa present.

DIAGNOSIS

Culture of the external auditory canal confirms the diagnosis of otitis externa. However, practically speaking, it is rarely obtained or needed. Because the primary sign of otitis externa is otorrhea, its differential diagnosis serves as that for otitis externa in general.

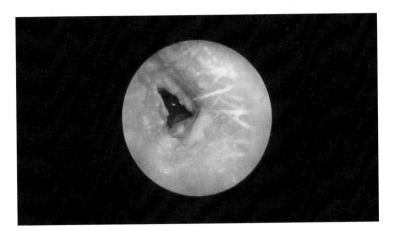

Figure 11–1 Acute diffuse otitis externa with erythema and swelling of the exernal auditory canal skin with scant otorrhea.

In the following types of otitis externa, otorrhea will have differing qualities:

- acute–bacterial: scanty white mucoid discharge (occasionally thick)
- chronic–bacterial: can be bloody; granulation tissue is often present
- fungal—white to off-white discharge, which may also be black, gray, bluish-green, or yellow. It can also present as black or white conidiophores on white hyphae associated with *Aspergillus*.

In otitis media with perforated tympanic membrane, otorrhea will have the following qualities:

- acute—purulent white to yellow mucus with deep pain
- serous—clear mucus, especially in the presence of allergies
- chronic—intermittent purulent mucus without pain
- cerebrospinal fluid leak—clear, thin, and watery discharge
- trauma—bloody mucus
- osteomyelitis—granulation tissue, discharge, and odor-imaging studies may be needed

CHAPTER 12

MANAGEMENT

This chapter outlines all of the known therapies for otitis externa. Before treatments are instituted, the area should be thoroughly cleaned, a culture taken when necessary, and pain relief administered.

AURAL TOILET

When otitis externa is diagnosed, the removal of as much debris as possible is crucial. This is best achieved with suction (with or without microscopy), but dry mopping or gentle curettage can be an alternative. Cotton-tipped applicators (other than for mopping out discharge around the meatal opening) are best avoided as they tend to push the debris further into the canal. "Tissue spears" twisted into a point and inserted into the canal about 2 cm and then allowed to absorb the discharge (and repeated as required) can help clear a watery discharge and obtain deeper access when medication is to be instilled.

If the external auditory canal is so swollen that topical therapy cannot be effectively delivered, a wick may be required (Figure 12-1). A wick serves to deliver the ototopical agent uniformly to the entire canal while also providing aural toilet if it is changed frequently. Additionally, it also allows for a depot delivery mechanism if dosing is frequent enough to keep the wick moist and continuously impregnated with the antibiotic. Although practices vary, changing the wick every 2 to 5 days with aural toilet is common practice. Wicks are underused, especially in the United States, not only in the treatment of otitis externa but also in the treatment of acute otitis media with otorrhea. There is no well-designed prospective trial proving this point in the published literature. The

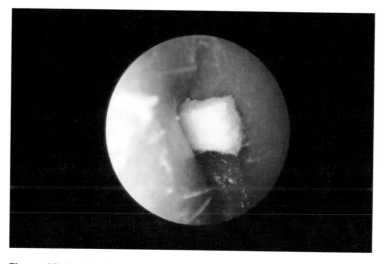

Figure 12–1 Nonfenestrated Pope otowick in acute diffuse otitis externa.

science is not of high enough impact to gain funding through the National Institutes of Health, and there is relatively little benefit to industry to fund such a trial. Also, in general, primary care physicians who care for the majority of uncomplicated cases are less experienced in otowick placement. This is one area that will hopefully become better studied and established in the future.

CULTURE

Culture and sensitivity are indicated if the patient fails initial outpatient therapy with an appropriate ototopical medication. A culture should also be obtained if the patient has high-risk comorbid factors such as immunodeficiency. Finally, if extension beyond the soft tissue of the external auditory canal or infection owing to an atypical pathogen is suspected, a culture should also be obtained. The sample should be taken from the more medial aspect of the canal under visualization to obviate sampling error, and a wire/cotton swab should be used to reduce secondary bacterial contaminants. Both bacterial and fungal stains and cultures should be obtained and, in selected cases, viral cultures as well. Although bacterial in vitro susceptibilities may not correlate with clinical outcomes because breakpoints are determined for systemic, not topical, administration, identifying the organism, and especially distinguishing a fungal from a bacterial infection, is of therapeutic significance.

ANALGESIA

Often overlooked, analgesia is an important adjunct to provide in the early course of otitis externa. The nature of the agent used depends on the severity of the pain. Fortunately, a wide range of medications are available to physicians for the treatment of earache. Ototopical anesthetics are available that contain antipyrine, glycerine, and benzocaine (Auralgan Otic Solution) and are effective in reducing ear pain in children with ear infections for milder cases (Hoberman, 1997). When pain is more severe, systemic agents such as aspirin, acetaminophen, codeine, ibuprofen, or prescription narcotics can be used. There are data to suggest that the addition of a corticosteroid to a topical quinolone expedites resolution of pain in otitis externa (Pistorius et al, 1999). Such a combination is presently available in the United States (CiproHC), and a second combination substituting a strong corticosteroid, dexamethasone, for hydrocortisone is in development (see in this chapter in the section on corticosteroids).

TREATMENTS

Infections of the ear, such as otitis externa, can cause debilitating pain, hearing loss, and discomfort. Over the centuries, imaginative approaches have been developed to treat these common and irritating infections.

Topical Treatments

Ancient treatments.   Ear candling.   Over the centuries, several creative approaches have been developed to treat otitis externa. One in particular, called ear candling, has been used for nearly 1,000 years in many diverse geographic locations, including North America, South America, China, and Egypt. This therapy involves placing a hollow candle into the external ear canal and lighting the opposite end, which is thought to create a vacuum that draws cerumen (ear wax), bacteria, and debris out of the ear (Seely et al, 1996). Ear candles are still used today by holistic and alternative health practitioners, but results from a clinical study suggest that this procedure is not effective and might actually be harmful. The study examined the ability of commercially available ear candles to generate a vacuum and to remove cerumen from eight ears; four of the eight ears had impacted cerumen (Seely et al, 1996). After 20 attempts with two different candle types, the generation of a vacuum could not be demonstrated with a device consisting of a two-chambered tube with a tympanometer probe inside each chamber. The ear candles also did not remove any noticeable cerumen from the four impacted ears, and the procedure actually deposited candle wax in two of the four ears that were originally free of excess cerumen.

Interestingly, results from a survey of otolaryngologists conducted by the authors revealed that one-third (40) of the responding physicians were aware of ear candling by one or more of their patients. In addition, 21 ear injuries were reported among 20 patients who were treated by these physicians for ear candle–induced complications. These injuries included burns, occlusions of the ear canal with candle wax, and a tympanic membrane perforation (Seely et al, 1996).

Topical astringents and alcohols. The topical application of various astringents and alcohols has also been used throughout history for ear infections (Myer, 2001). Those that were acidic or contained high concentrations of alcohol may have been effective if they were administered early in the disease (Sander, 2001). In fact, certain astringents, such as boric acid and aluminum acetate, are considered effective and are sometimes used today (Clayton et al, 1990; Slack, 1987). The disadvantages of using these treatments are that they may not have adequate antimicrobial activity to eradicate pathogens in moderate to severe cases and are painful to the patient, which may affect compliance.

Topical acetic acid. Solutions containing acetic acid are often used today to prevent and treat mild to moderate cases of otitis externa (Sander, 2001). These "antiseptics" were a main component in the management of ear infections before the discovery of antibiotics. Solutions containing acetic acid have in vitro antimicrobial activity against the common pathogens of otitis externa (*Pseudomonas aeruginosa* and *Staphylococcus aureus*) and are effective in several types of ear infections, including otitis externa, otitis media, and granular myringitis (Aminifarshidmehr, 1996; Sander, 2001; Thorp et al, 1998). Their efficacy is based on their ability to reduce the pH in the ear. Low pH restricts the growth of bacteria and fungi, which flourish in a basic environment (pH 8–10) (Aminifarshidmehr, 1996).

Solutions containing acetic acid have disadvantages despite their ability to resolve ear infections. For example, they are painful to the patient because they irritate inflamed skin. This may have a negative influence on patient compliance because they are often required to be administered multiple times per day (Otic Domeboro package insert, 1995). Also, otic drops containing acetic acid have the potential to cause ototoxicity if they gain access to the inner ear. In a recent study, acetic acid was found to cause more damage to isolated cochlear outer hair cells compared with otic treatments containing antibiotics (Jinn et al, 2001). This is a genuine concern because resolution of ear infections with acetic acid may require long treatment periods (3 weeks), which increases the likelihood of ototoxicity. Acidification may be necessary for maintenance if cerumen production is absent after resolution of the infection or as prophylaxis in recurrent cases, especially in patients with risk factors that alter the physiologic pH of the external auditory canal, such as swimming.

Ototopical Treatments

Understanding the pathogenesis of otitis externa is basic to the development of efficacious therapies. Several of the early modern treatments for this disease inhibited the growth of both bacteria and fungi simply because they were acidic. In contrast, the newer topical antibiotic treatments, although highly effective against bacteria-induced disease, have no or limited antifungal activity. Over time, treatments for otitis externa have evolved into therapies that have predominantly antibacteriologic activity, low potential for ototoxicity, and convenient dosing regimens.

Topical versus Systemic Therapy

Currently, topical antibiotics are the most common therapy prescribed by physicians for the treatment of otitis externa (Halpern et al, 1999; Rowlands et al, 2001). However, in spite of educational efforts to the contrary, many physicians continue to treat otitis externa with systemic rather than topical antibiotics. There are many advantages to using topical rather than systemic therapy:

Topical medications are delivered directly to the target organ. Compared with oral antibiotics, topical antibiotics are more effective and have been shown to result in lower disease persistence rates and recurrence rates (Rowlands et al, 2001). This is because topical antibiotics are applied directly to the bacteria in the ear at concentrations well over the minimum inhibitory concentration (MIC) needed for pathogen eradication (Cipro HC Otic package insert, 2002; Cortisporin Otic Suspension Sterile package insert, 2000; Floxin Otic package insert, 1999; Hooper, 2000; Roland and Stroman, 2002). A recent study by Ohyama and colleagues (1999) found that drug concentrations of the topical antibiotic ofloxacin otic (Floxin Otic) can remain above the MIC for *S. aureus* in otorrhea samples for up to 8 hours in some patients. By bypassing the systemic circulation, pharmacokinetic factors such as solubility, intestinal absorption, and hepatic first-pass effects do not affect ultimate tissue concentrations. Importantly, in the same study, serum testing indicated that drug concentrations were below the limit of detection in most of the serum samples, which indicates that this antibiotic is not efficiently absorbed into the systemic circulation. This is advantageous because it maintains high drug concentrations at the site of infection and lessens the potential for systemic adverse effects.

Topical antibiotics do not lead to the development of resistance. The US Food and Drug Administration (FDA) has stated that it ". . . is unaware of any evidence that . . . topical antibiotics . . . have led to an increase in infection in the general population by resistant organisms . . . The agency believes that if resistance were a problem . . . it would have been known by now" (Langford and Benrimoj, 1996). This tenet on resistance and topical therapy holds for short-term use, provided that drug delivery is effective. This point was corroborated by a study done in Pittsburgh. Two hundred thirty-one consecutive children presenting to the outpatient otolaryngology clinic with draining ears from which *P. aeruginosa* was isolated were studied (Dohar et al, 1996). Of these, 99.6% showed a sensitivity to polymyxin B, one of the active ingredients in Cortisporin Otic Suspension, used very commonly in the community since the 1970s. Only one strain of *P. aeruginosa* proved resistant to polymyxin B. The authors concluded that despite widespread use of ototopical Cortisporin Otic Suspension for nearly three decades, *P. aeruginosa* remained sensitive to it. This failure to invoke resistance has been observed for topical skin antibiotics and topical eye drops. It is likely that the reason for this is because the concentrations of topical antibiotics exceed the MICs at the site of infection to such a degree that eradication is more rapid and complete.

Also, topical therapy is generally used in relatively short treatment courses. When reports of resistance to a topical agent are made, a critical reviewer must carefully examine them to search for a reason. For example, a recent report by Berenholz and colleagues (2002) concluded that an increased resistance to ciprofloxacin (CiproHC) by *P. aeruginosa* was observed in a select population of patients with otitis externa. The key here is that this is an agent in common use systemically and its systemic, not ototopical, use is likely that responsible for the emergence of increased resistance.

Another common explanation for reports citing emergence of bacterial resistance to topical antibiotics is inadequate drug delivery. This has been the case in lower respiratory and sinus infections. Generally speaking, this should not be the case in middle ear infections. It is important to note that all five significant pathogens most commonly isolated from draining ears, *P. aeruginosa*, *Streptococcus pneumonia*, *S. aureus*, *Haemophilus influenzae, and Moraxella catarrhalis*, are of major concern owing to their propensity to develop resistance. This fact, coupled with the relatively high prevalence of otitis media and the substantial public health concern that the issue of bacterial resistance has become, strongly supports the development of strategies to minimize resistance from developing in the future.

Topical strategies have a lower incidence of adverse events. The product label of systemic antibiotics lists such common side effects as diarrhea, nausea, rash, vomiting, abdominal pain, and headache, along with more severe side effects such as Stevens-Johnson syndrome, aplastic anemia, seizure, and anaphylaxis. With the newer topical agents, only minor local irritative and allergic effects are seen—a marked advantage. A recent trial comparing the efficacy and safety of topical ofloxacin with amoxicillin and clavulanate found an incidence of 6% treatment-related side effects associated with the ototopical agent compared with 31% for the systemic agent (Goldblatt et al, 1998). The improved safety profile of topical over systemic antimicrobials is unequivocal.

A higher incidence of adverse events has been reported for older ototopical agents. Most of these were local sensitivity responses and were most frequently seen with products containing neomycin. The major disadvantage of neomycin is its propensity to lead to sensitization. This manifests as allergic inflammation, most often of the skin of the external auditory canal and pinna. Van Ginkel and colleagues (1995) stated that "Because of the high risk of sensitization, topical preparations containing neomycin . . . should not be used routinely." In patients with otitis externa who have been treated topically, neomycin is invariably the most important sensitizer (Fraki et al, 1985; Holmes et al, 1982; Pigatto et al, 1991; Rasmussen, 1974; Smith et al, 1990). Neomycin sensitization is vastly underestimated. When used in the external auditory canal, the package insert states that the manifestation of sensitization to neomycin is usually a low-grade reddening with swelling, dry scaling, and itching (*Physician's Desk Reference*, 1995). It may manifest as failure to heal. Given the experience in nasal allergy, we know that mucosa responds to allergic triggers with edema and drainage. Clearly, in both skin and mucosa, the inflammatory manifestations of allergy and infection are clinically similar, if not indistinguishable.

Topical antibiotics have withstood the test of time but continue to evolve. Otic treatments containing aminoglycoside antibiotics have been available for over 20 years and are still widely prescribed. These drugs are usually combined with topical corticosteroids and other antibiotics and are efficacious against otitis externa caused by bacteria. At the same time, newer oral antibiotics are being developed into topical treatments for ear infections. Otic formulations of fluoroquinolone antibiotics are the latest development in topical antibiotic therapy for otitis externa and are effective as monotherapy for the treatment of this disease.

In clinical settings, treatment preferences for otitis externa are currently evolving as physicians become concerned about adverse effects caused by the older antibiotic treatments and aware of newer options. The result has been a slow but steady replacement of the older antibiotic treatments with the newer topical antibiotics. Certain topical antibiotics are approved by the FDA for use against *P. aeruginosa* in children. In contrast, no oral antibiotics have been approved for this organism in children.

Corticosteroids

The need for a corticosteroid has become one of the most debated topics in the treatment of ear infections. The rationale for including a corticosteroid in ototopical preparations is theoretically sound. Corticosteroids have known, potent, anti-inflammatory activity. Because ototopical agents are most commonly used in conditions of the ear in which inflammation is a prominent component (most often as a result of infection), including a corticosteroid seems reasonable.

An exhaustive review of all issues relating to corticosteroid formulation and use is beyond the scope of this text. What is reviewed is a summary of the considerations important in selecting a corticosteroid (most often a topical formulation) for otic inflammatory conditions, as well as a brief review of the clinical data on corticosteroid use, both pro and con, available for otitis externa.

Selecting a corticosteroid. Corticosteroids may differ in formulation and potency, and both can effect clinical outcomes. Thus, a fine line exists between choosing a corticosteroid that is more potent to expedite the resolution of inflammation but not so potent that safety is compromised either by local immune suppression, tissue toxicity, or increased systemic absorption, leading to the well-understood consequence of adrenal axis suppression.

Although it does not follow that "more potent" corticosteroids used topically result in higher serum concentrations, it is certain that higher solubility and tissue concentrations in the target tissue (ie, the middle ear mucosa) are directly proportional to ultimate serum concentrations. This presents yet another issue of using an agent not only "potent enough" but also "soluble enough" to achieve an optimal clinical anti-inflammatory outcome. Yet one does not want a corticosteroid "so soluble" that substantial serum levels result or "so potent" that local toxic effects result. The good news in using topical corticosteroids in inflammatory ear disease is that, by and large, the treatment courses are relatively short, thus obviating the significant adverse effects of systemic absorption. There are some chronic inflammatory diseases of the ear, however, for which topical corticosteroids may be necessary in longer, "off-label" courses, and, in these cases, such issues must be considered. Lastly, although both hydrocortisone and dexamethasone have traditionally been classified in conversion tables as "low potency," in topical formulations, this is absolutely untrue, with dexamethasone showing clear superiority.

Review of clinical data. Many are under the misconception that the addition of a corticosteroid "may help but cannot hurt." This is not entirely true. The 49th edition of the *Physician's Desk Reference* (1995) states in a warning for Cortisporin that, "Since corticoids may inhibit the body's defense mechanism against infection, a concomitant antimicrobial drug may be used when this inhibition is considered to be clinically significant in a particular case." Additionally, we think of corticosteroids as anti-inflammatory agents, yet the opposite can be observed. Van Ginkel and colleagues (1995) explained that "In spite of their intrinsic anti-inflammatory activity, topical steroids can also enhance the inflammation due to sensitization." They demonstrated that 6 of 34 patients (18%) with chronic otorrhea (ie, > 3 months) treated with a corticosteroid-containing ototopical agent had patch tests positive to corticosteroids. This is particularly concerning for two reasons. First, it causes one to wonder if those patients with chronic inflammatory ear conditions who are refractory and have been treated with a corticosteroid-containing topical agent may, in fact, be experiencing allergic inflammation perpetuated by continued exposure to the corticosteroid. Second, physicians use corticosteroids for protracted lengths of time to treat other common diseases, such as asthma and rhinitis. Are we compounding allergic sensitization in susceptible patients with overuse? At present, there is no evidence-based answer to this question.

There are few studies providing evidence-based support for using topical corticosteroids to treat otitis externa. The best clinical trial favoring corticosteroids compared ciprofloxacin alone with ciprofloxacin plus hydrocortisone to treat otitis externa. The results revealed a more rapid time to pain resolution (0.8 days) when the corticosteroid was added to the fluoroquinolone compared with treatment with the fluoroquinolone alone (Pistorius et al, 1998).

Other clinical trials brought into question the need for a combination corticosteroid/antibiotic in all cases. The safety and efficacy of Floxin Otic solution were compared with those of Cortisporin Otic solution (neomycin sulfate, polymyxin B sulfate, and hydrocortisone) in the treatment of otitis externa in children and adults (Jones et al, 1997). The trials were of reasonable sample size, enrolling 314 adults and 287 children, respectively. The investigators found no statistically significant differences in clinical outcomes or eradication rates for *P. aeruginosa* and *S. aureus*. Discomfort was assessed by each subject and parent or guardian, and the data were culled from the submitted diaries. There was no difference in time to cessation of pain. These data would suggest that there was no added benefit of the corticosteroid/hydrocortisone combined with the anti-infectives in Cortisporin compared with Floxin Otic alone, which does not contain a corticosteroid.

Three questions arise from these trials. First, the comparison was not ideal: using the same antibiotic with or without the corticosteroid would have provided a more straightforward comparison. However, using Cortisporin as one of the comparitors was appropriate because Cortisporin was the most widely used drug to treat otitis externa at the time of the trial. Second, and more importantly, if the trial had used a more sophisticated pain scale, rather than diary data, would there have been a difference in time to resolution of pain? Third, would a more potent corticosteroid, such as dexamethasone, have effected different outcomes? Further study is necessary to resolve these questions. Until then, the rationale for using a combination topical agent of antibiotic and corticosteroid (eg, CiproHC, Ciprodex) is sound, and one clinical trial demonstrated clear benefit. The disadvantages of using topical corticosteroids in the external ear canal are not generally appreciated in association with short courses of therapy. Safety and more convenient dosing schedules favor the more recently developed quinolone/corticosteroid formulations (CiproHC) over older ones (eg, Cortosporin Otic Solution). It is likely that the efficacy of products currently in development (Ciprodex) will prove superior to older ones, although the data are not yet published.

Multiple Antimicrobial Agents

Some treatments contain more than one antimicrobial agent in any single formulation. Cortisporin, Pediotic Suspension, and Coly-Mycin are all examples of preparations that contain one or more antibiotics. The rationale for the combination of antibiotics in these preparations is unclear.

Polymyxin B sulfate (10,000 U/mL), represented in most topical ear preparations, is effective against *P. aeruginosa* and other gram-negative bacteria, including strains of *Escherichia* (*Physician's Desk Reference*, 1988). Similarly, colistin sulfate (3 mg/mL) is effective against most gram-negative organisms, notably *P. aeruginosa*, *Escherichia coli*, and *Klebsiella* species (Jackman et al, 2002). Neomycin sulfate (3.3 mg/mL) is an aminoglycoside, again with primary effectiveness against many gram-negative organisms and some activity against *S. aureus*.

Surprisingly, from an anti-infective perspective, it is the activity against the gram-positive staphylococci that probably led to the inclusion of neomycin, activity not generally emphasized for antibiotics belonging to the aminoglycoside class. The other possible rationale for the inclusion of neomycin was to provide a second antibiotic to act synergistically with polymyxin B against *Pseudomonas*. It has traditionally been taught that "dual" antibiotic therapy is necessary when treating *Pseudomonas* infections causing pneumonia or infection in immunocompromised patients (Menzies and Gregory, 1996). This premise has been based on the rationale that the synergy of two drugs with different modes of activity reduces the likelihood of treatment-induced resistance and more effectively eradicates the organism.

The data on the treatment of aural *Pseudomonas* infections have not supported the need for dual therapy. A study from Pittsburgh revealed excellent in vitro susceptibility of aural isolates of *P. aeruginosa* to the semisynthetic penicillins. Single-agent intravenous therapy from this class of antibiotics has been the standard treatment for chronic suppurative otitis media owing to *P. aeruginosa* in children, refractory to outpatient management, with excellent results (Dohar et al, 1995).

The fluoroquinolones, as mentioned previously, achieve the appropriate coverage of both the gram-positive and gram-negative bacterial pathogens commonly recovered from draining ears.

Other Components

When evaluating systemic drugs, most of the emphasis is on the active ingredients of the formulation. Although this way of thinking spills over to the evaluation of topical agents, one must resist the temptation to ignore other components of the formulation, but they are important in several ways. First, vehicular components may possess antimicrobial activity either primarily or synergistically in combination with other compounds. Second, vehicular components may contribute as significantly or even more significantly to the side-effect profile of the compound. Third, the biocompatibility of the drug may be heavily influenced by these components.

Components of the vehicle may act opposite to the desired clinical outcome. For example, many older ototopical formulations contained propylene glycol. This is one of the compounds sold as antifreeze. Although seemingly irrelevant, there is a considerable irritative effect on the tissue by such a compound. Barlow and colleagues (1994) found that Cortisporin Otic Suspension produced moderate to severe middle ear musocal thickening, moderate periosteal thickening, and inflammatory cell infiltration and resultant thickening of the tympanic membrane. Similar effects might be expected in the skin of the external auditory canal, although this has not been systematically studied.

More recent attention has been given to the excipient preservatives of newer topical agents. Most of the research has focused on topical intranasal corticosteroids, although there is little reason to believe that a significant difference would exist between middle ear and nasal mucosa or possibly even the skin of the external auditory canal. Benzalkonium chloride (BKC) is the most widely used preservative in topical nasal corticosteroids and newer ototopical preparations such as Floxin Otic. It may also be found in ophthalmic, pulmonary, and dermatologic topical products as well. It is a quaternary ammonium compound first introduced in 1935 as an antiseptic agent. Such mucosal changes as squamous metaplasia, loss of cilia, loss of goblet cells, and a lack of mucus covering the epithelium have been observed (Berg et al, 1997). Ciliostasis was promoted, and a reduction in mucociliary transport was measured. Reflex mucosal congestion was also noted with long-term use. Additionally, systemic reactions to topical exposures such as hypersensitivity lung syndrome with circulating immune complexes were seen. As an aside, BKC found in most Dutch ototopical preparations hardly elicited any allergic reaction at all, with 1 of 34 patients demonstrating a positive skin test to it (van Ginkel et al, 1995). Polyvinyl alcohol is yet another preservative found in more recent ototopical preparations (CiproHC). Anecdotes of polymerization of this substance leading to obstructed tympanostomy tubes and cast formation within the external auditory canal have been discussed. Although suspected to be, in part, a function of higher than recommended dosages or longer than recommended treatment courses, neither mechanism explained some cases. The concentration of polyvinyl alcohol has been reduced in the current formulation of CiproHC to prevent this complication in the future. Although it is likely that preservative effects such as those described above are reversible when a short treatment course (less than 14 days) is prescribed, longer off-label use may present a variety of problems, with those attributable to the preservative being among them. Future research efforts are focusing on compounds with intrinsic properties, obviating the need for a preservative. Until such products are available, judicious use of such agents must be practiced.

Systemic Antibiotics

Systemic antibiotics are rarely needed. Generally, they are used only when otitis externa is persistent, associated otitis media is present, or local or systemic spread has occurred beyond the external auditory canal. Spread is suspected if the temperature is above 38.3°C or pain is out of proportion to clinical findings. Systemic antibiotics should also be considered in high-risk patients such as diabetic patients or immunocompromised hosts.

SURGERY

Surgery is rarely required but may be necessary in cases of necrotizing otitis externa, wherein devitalized sequestrations of bone may need to be débrided. In cases of a very narrow external auditory canal secondary to grossly hypertrophic canal skin, surgery may also be indicated to optimize the anatomy. Swimmer's exotoses can predispose to otitis externa and may require surgical removal (Figure 12-2).

PREVENTION

Prevention of recurrence of otitis externa primarily consists of avoiding predisposing factors and treating underlying dermatologic conditions. Swimming should be avoided until the infection resolves, and dry ear precautions should be instituted. Acidifying drops may be beneficial, as mentioned previously. Patients should avoid any trauma to the external auditory canal, such as scratching or overzealous cleaning. Topical corticosteroids may be of considerable benefit in reducing residual pruritus.

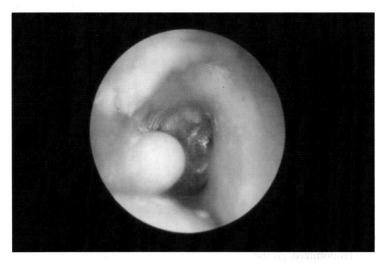

Figure 12–2 Exotoses of the external auditory canal potentially predisposing to otitis externa.

CONCLUSION

The availability of the otic fluoroquinolones has allowed physicians to re-evaluate treatment options for otitis externa. This has led to a steady shift in treatment preference from the older combination drugs to ofloxacin and ciprofloxacin. This recent evolution in management is based on differences in treatment characteristics. Physicians are seeing an increase in the incidence of adverse effects, such as hypersensitivity, with drugs containing neomycin and polymyxin B. Also, physicians would rather not risk the possibility of ototoxicity that is associated with these older drugs. Topical ofloxacin and ciprofloxacin are now the preferred treatments, in part because adverse effects with these drugs have been rare in otitis externa. Physicians also appreciate the influence of the vehicle on patient health, such as hypersensitivity or irritation toward vehicle components (eg, thimerosal, propylene glycol).

REFERENCES

Aminifarshidmehr N. The management of chronic suppurative otitis media with acid media solution. Am J Otol 1996;17:24–5.

Barlow DW, Duckert LG, Kreig SC, Gates GA. Ototoxicity of topical otomicrobial agents. Acta Otolaryngol (Stockh) 1994;115:231–5.

Berenholz L, Katzenell U, Harell M. Evolving resistant *Pseudomonas* to ciprofloxacin in malignant otitis externa. Laryngoscope 2002;112: 1619–22.

Berg OH, Lie K, Steinsvag SK. The effects of topical nasal steroids on rat respiratory mucosa in vitro, with special reference to benzalkonium chloride. Allergy 1997;52:627–32.

Cipro HC Otic [package insert]. Fort Worth (TX): Alcon Laboratories, Inc.; 2002.

Clayton MI, Osborne JE, Rutherford D, Rivron RP. A double-blind, randomized, prospective trial of a topical antiseptic versus a topical antibiotic in the treatment of otorrhoea. Clin Otolaryngol 1990; 15:7–10.

Cortisporin Otic Suspension Sterile [package insert]. Greenville (NC): Catalytica Pharmaceuticals, Inc.; 2000.

Dohar JE, Kenna MA, Wadowsky RM. In vitro susceptibility of aural isolates of *P. aeruginosa* to commonly used ototopical antibiotics. Am J Otol 1996;17:207–9.

Dohar JE, Kenna MA, Wadowsky RM. Therapeutic implications in the treatment of aural *Pseudomonas* infections based on in vitro susceptibility patterns. Arch Otolaryngol Head Neck Surg 1995;121: 1022–5.

Floxin Otic [package insert]. Montvale (NJ): Daiichi Pharmaceutical Corporation; 1999.

Fraki JE, Kalimo K, Tuohimaa P, Aantaa E. Contact allergy to various components of topical preparations for treatment of external otitis. Acta Otolaryngol (Stockh) 1985;100:414–8.

Goldblatt EL, Dohar JE, Nozza RJ, et al. Topical ofloxacin versus systemic amoxicillin/clavulanate in purulent otorrhea in children with tympanostomy tubes. Int J Pediatr Otorhinolaryngol 1998;46: 91–101.

Halpern MT, Palmer CS, Seidlin M. Treatment patterns for otitis externa. J Am Board Fam Pract 1999;12:1–7.

Hoberman A, Paradise JL, Reynolds EA, Urkin J. Efficacy of Auralgan for treating ear pain in children with acute otitis media. Arch Pediatr Adolesc Med 1997;151:675–8.

Holmes RC, Johns AN, Wilkinson JD, et al. Medicament contact dermatitis in patients with chronic inflammatory disease. J R Soc Med 1982;75:27–30.

Hooper DC. Quinolones. In: Mandell G, Bennett J, Dolin R, editors. Mandell, Douglas, and Bennett's principles and practice of infectious diseases. 5th ed. Philadelphia: Churchill Livingstone; 2000. p. 404–13.

Jackman A, Bent J, April M, Ward R. Topical antibiotics induced otomycosis [abstract]. In: American Society of Pediatric Otolaryngology Seventeenth Annual Meeting, Boca Raton, FL, May 11–14, 2002.

Jinn TH, Kim PD, Russell PT, et al. Determination of ototoxicity of common otic drops using isolated cochlear outer hair cells. Laryngoscope 2001;111:2105–8.

Langford JH, Benrimoj SI. Clinical rationale for topical antimicrobial preparations. J Antimicrob Chemother 1996;37:399–402.

Menzies B, Gregory DW. *Pseudomonas*. In: Schlossberg D, editor. Current therapy of infectious disease. St. Louis: Mosby-Year Book; 1996. p. 446–50.

Myer CMI. Historical perspective on the use of otic antimicrobial agents. Pediatr Infect Dis J 2001;20:98–101.

Ohyama M, Furuta S, Ueno K, et al. Ofloxacin otic solution in patients with otitis media: an analysis of drug concentrations. Arch Otolaryngol Head Neck Surg 1999;125:337–40.

Otic Domeboro [package Insert]. West Haven (CT): Bayer Corporation; 1995.

Physician's desk reference. 42nd ed. Montvale (NJ): Medical Economics Data Production Company; 1988.

Physician's desk reference. 49th ed. Montvale (NJ): Medical Economics Data Production Company; 1995.

Pigatto PD, Bigardi A, Legori A, et al. Allergic contact dermatitis prevalence in patients with otitis externa. Acta Derm Venereol 1991;71: 162–5.

Pistorius B, Westberry K, Drehobl M, et al. Prospective, randomized, comparative trial of ciprofloxacin otic drops, with or without hydrocortisone vs. polymyxin B-neomycin-hydrocortisone otic suspension in the treatment of acute diffuse otitis externa. Infect Dis Clin Pract 1999;8:387–95.

Rasmussen PA. Otitis externa and allergic contact dermatitis. Acta Otolaryngol (Stockh) 1974;77:344–7.

Roland PS, Stroman DW. Microbiology of acute otitis externa. Laryngoscope 2002;112:1166–77.

Rowlands S, Devalia H, Smith C, et al. Otitis externa in UK general practice: a survey using the UK General Practice Research Database. Br J Gen Pract 2001;51:533–8.

Sander R. Otitis externa: a practical guide to treatment and prevention. Am Fam Physician 2001;63:927–36.

Seely DR, Quigley SM, Langman AW. Ear candles—efficacy and safety. Laryngoscope 1996;106:1226–9.

Slack RW. A study of three preparations in the treatment of otitis externa. J Laryngol Otol 1987;101:533–5.

Smith IM, Keay DG, Buxton PK. Contact hypersensitivity in patients with chronic otitis externa. Clin Otolaryngol 1990;15: 155–8.

Thorp MA, Kruger J, Oliver S, et al. The antibacterial activity of acetic acid and Burow's solution as topical otological preparations. J Laryngol Otol 1998;112:925–8.

van Ginkel CJ, Bruintjes TD, Huizing EH. Allergy due to topical medications in chronic otitis externa and chronic otitis media. Clin Otolaryngol 1995;20:326–8.

CHAPTER 13

FUTURE DIRECTIONS FOR OTITIS MEDIA AND OTITIS EXTERNA

Research into the epidemiology, etiology, pathogenesis, and management of otitis media and otitis externa is ongoing. It is hoped that this research will ultimately bring major advances in the understanding of these diseases and more safe and effective methods to treat and prevent them.

OTITIS MEDIA

Because we know that there is a genetic predisposition for otitis media (Casselbrant et al, 1999), we are currently engaged in searching for the genes that may be underlying causative factors. This research is being funded by the National Institutes of Health (NIH); it is hoped that within the next several years we may have more insight into why the disease seems to "run in families." Also with NIH funding, we are investigating the following:

- the role of virus and genetic susceptibility to otitis media
- the role of biofilms (the coating around certain bacteria, such as *Pseudomonas*) in the pathogenesis of otorrhea
- normal and abnormal gas composition of the middle ear
- the role that eustachian tube dysfunction plays in recurrent and chronic disease and methods to normalize this dysfunction
- the effect of middle ear effusion on balance function
- the efficacy of inflation of the middle ear (modified Politzer's method) in clearing middle ear effusions
- the efficacy of surgery (myringotomy with tympanostomy tube insertion, adenoidectomy) in young children who have chronic otitis media with effusion

Many investigators are concentrating on otitis media to develop new safe and effective vaccines for prevention of the viruses that cause the common cold because they initiate most episodes of acute otitis media. Also, drugs are under investigation to abate an upper respiratory infection, which may help prevent otitis media. Even though we have a vaccine that is highly effective in preventing *Haemophilus influenzae* type b infections, which only cause a small percentage of otitis media, we currently do not have a vaccine for prevention of nontypeable *H. influenzae*, which still causes approximately 25% of acute middle ear infections. Unfortunately, even though the new conjugate pneumococcal vaccine (Prevnar) is highly effective in preventing pneumococcal meningitis, it has limited success in preventing pneumococcal otitis media (see the section on recurrent acute otitis media in Chapter 7, "Management"). Also, *Moraxella catarrhalis* is the cause of about 15% of acute otitis media, but we currently do not have a vaccine for this bacterium. It is hoped that these vaccines will be available in the near future.

Even though a host of antimicrobial agents have been proven to be safe and effective for treatment of otitis media in the past, the bacterial organisms have become increasingly resistant to many of them, leaving us with few and fewer options that are still effective. Fortunately, industry is trying to keep pace. One class of antimicrobial agents, the quinolones, offers an attractive new addition to our treatment options, especially when *Pseudomonas* is the causative organism. However, as a systemic agent, they are not currently approved for children under the age of 17 years, but we may have approved systemic quinolone agents in the near future. Fortunately, we have topical quinolone agents (FloxinOtic, CiproDex) that are approved for treatment of otorrhea, and we anticipate that future ototopical agents will become available to treat acute and chronic otorrhea.

Some nontraditional methods to prevent otitis media have showed some promise in clinical trials. Oligosaccharides and xylitol appear to prevent experimental pneumococcal attachment to respiratory mucosa, but more evidence is needed before being recommended for clinical use.

OTITIS EXTERNA

The future direction for otitis externa centers on the continuing quest to eradicate the pathogens responsible for the infection and to reduce the associated ear pain.

The treatment objectives for otitis externa have remained consistent, whereas treatment approaches have evolved. As just stated, the main goal of therapy is to eradicate the pathogens responsible for the infection, commonly *Pseudomonas aeruginosa* and *Staphylococcus aureus* (Agius et al, 1992; Hawke et al, 1984).

In some geographic areas, *S. aureus* is becoming more common than *P. aeruginosa*, and the prevalence of community-acquired methicillin-resistant *S. aureus* infections in discharging ears is also increasing (Hwang et al, 2002). Needless to say, eradication is most efficiently achieved with antibiotics that have antimicrobial activity against these pathogens.

In the not too distant past, topical solutions containing acids and alcohols were common therapies for the treatment of ear infections. Treatment preferences changed when topical corticosteroids and antibiotics became readily available in the latter half of the twentieth century. However, only a handful of antibiotics have been developed into topical treatments specifically for ear infections such as otitis externa. For the past 20 years, combination drugs containing an aminoglycoside, polymyxin B, and a corticosteroid have been the main topical antibiotic treatments available to treat ear infections.

This period of inactivity in topical antibiotic development ended approximately 5 years ago when newer oral antibiotics belonging to the fluoroquinolone class of antimicrobial agents were formulated into topical treatments for ear infections. This research push was fueled by concern about the potential for adverse effects caused by the older combination antibiotic treatments and the desire among physicians to prescribe therapies that favor patient compliance and are unlikely to cause ototoxicity. The availability of these newer otic therapies allows physicians to rethink their treatment strategies for otitis externa. The result has been an evolution in treatment preference from the older combination drugs toward the newer fluoroquinolone otic therapies.

Another objective of treatment in addition to eradicating the infectious pathogens is reducing ear pain. Earache is a common and significant symptom of otitis externa, and its intensity is directly related to disease severity (Agius et al, 1992; Hawke et al, 1984). In fact, not uncommonly, pain results in the discontinuation of daily activities or bed rest (van Asperen et al, 1995). The treatment of pain was outlined previously in Chapter 12, "Management," in the section on analgesia.

REFERENCES

Agius AM, Pickles JM, Burch KL. A prospective study of otitis externa. Clin Otolaryngol 1992;17:150–4.

Casselbrant ML, Mandel EM, Fall PA, et al. The heritability of otitis media: a twin/triplet study. JAMA 1999;282:2125–30.

Hawke M, Wong J, Krajden S. Clinical and microbiological features of otitis externa. J Otolaryngol 1984;13:289–95.

Hwang J-H, Chu C-K, Liu T-C. Changes in bacteriology of discharging ears. J Laryngol Otol 2002;116:686–9.

van Asperen I, de Rover CM, Schijven JF, et al. Risk of otitis externa after swimming in recreational fresh water lakes containing *Pseudomonas aeruginosa*. BMJ 1995;311:1407–10.

The following is a glossary of commonly used terms related to otitis media and otitis externa. Many of these terms are used in this book.

Acute bacterial otitis externa is the medical term for swimmer's ear. It is one type of otitis externa.

Acute mastoiditis is a condition that occurs when a middle ear infection spreads to the mastoid. Signs include the outer ear pushing forward, swelling, tenderness, redness, and pain behind the outer ear. It is the most common complication of acute otitis media.

Acute otitis media is the rapid onset of signs and symptoms (such as earache, fever, and liquid in the middle ear) of acute infection in the middle ear.

Adenoidectomy is surgical removal of the adenoids.

Adenoids are a collection of lymphoid tissue behind the nose, similar to tonsils in the throat and glands (nodes) in the neck. Lymphoid tissue fights off infection.

Allergy is a potential cause of otitis media. Allergy symptoms include repeated sneezing spells, especially around freshly cut grass, dogs, or cats or during spring or fall; itching of the nose, eyes, and throat under the same circumstances; and a chronic runny nose.

Anatomic deformities are abnormalities of normal anatomy, such as a cleft palate. These can be a cause of recurring middle ear infections.

Antibiotic prophylaxis is giving a low dose of an antibiotic every day as a preventive measure.

Antibiotics are drugs used to fight infections. They are grouped into families that make up their composition (the penicillins, the cephalosporins, etc). Antibiotics usually have a *generic name* (the name for their chemical composition) and a *trade name* (the name the manufacturer has given them). Some antibiotics do not have a trade name because they are available in generic form from several manufacturers, such as amoxicillin.

Antihistamine is a medication to treat allergies.

Anti-inflammatory medicines (such as a corticosteroid) are contained in many of the antibiotic ear drops that your doctor will probably prescribe for swimmer's ear. Anti-inflammatory medicines make swelling go down.

Audiogram is a graph made to show hearing. An **audiometer** is used to obtain an audiogram.

Bacteria are types of microorganisms. A bacterium is a single species. Common ones that are involved in otitis media are *Streptococcus pneumoniae, Haemophilus influenzae, Moraxella catarrhalis, Pseudomonas aeruginosa, Streptococcus pyogenes,* and *Staphylococcus aureus.* **Bacteria** also cause most cases of swimmer's ear. The bacteria that usually cause swimmer's ear are *P. aeruginosa* (60%), *S. aureus* (15 to 30%), and streptococci and *Proteus* species (all other cases). Bacteria that cause middle ear infections are *S. pneumoniae, H. influenzae,* and *M. catarrhalis.*

Barotitis is a buildup of fluid in the middle ear following barotrauma.

Barotrauma is injury to the middle ear caused by rapid changes in barometric pressure.

β**-Lactamase** is an enzyme produced by some bacteria that acts by "breaking" the part of the antibiotic that is designed to attack it.

Brain abscess is an enclosed pocket of pus inside the brain.

Cholesteatoma is a cyst-like structure in the middle ear (and sometimes in the mastoid) filled with cheesy, skin-like material.

Chronic eczematous otitis externa occurs when the outer ear is inflamed but not because of an infection. It is one type of otitis externa.

Chronic otitis media with effusion is otitis media with effusion that lasts for several months or longer. It is also called **glue ear** or **secretory otitis media**.

Chronic suppurative otitis media occurs when an ear drains for a number of weeks or months and there is a perforation (or tympanostomy tube) in the eardrum.

Cilia are tiny, hair-like structures in the lining of the eustachian tube and part of the middle ear that move toward the nose and help move unwanted secretions and organisms out of the eustachian tube and middle ear.

Cleft palate is a congenital, anatomic deformity of the palate in which the palate is open.

Cochlea is the hearing part of the inner ear (labyrinth).

Cochlear implant is a device—similar to but not a hearing aid—for profoundly deaf children and adults.

Complication is a condition that occurs during an illness.

Conductive hearing loss is caused by damage to the ear's conducting system: the outer ear and middle ear.

Decongestant is medication that can lessen symptoms of nasal congestion.

Ear wax is in all ears and keeps harmful substances from getting in. When water—especially underwater swimming or diving—causes the wax to come out, bacteria already in the ear that do not normally cause an infection can cause one.

Ear wick is a material that can expand when placed in the ear and appears more like a sponge that fills the ear canal.

Eardrum (also called the **tympanic membrane**) is the membrane that separates the middle ear from the ear canal and transmits sound to the hearing bones (ossicles).

Eustachian tube connects the back of the nose to the middle ear and serves mainly to ventilate, protect, and drain the middle ear.

Eustachian tube dysfunction is an abnormality of the eustachian tube that affects any or all of the tube's normal functions of ventilating, protecting, and draining the middle ear.

External ear canal is another name for the outer ear. Otitis externa mostly affects the external ear canal.

Facial paralysis involves the facial nerve that passes through the middle ear (and mastoid) and can occur during an attack of acute otitis media, especially in infants.

Feruncle is an outer ear infection in which only part of the ear canal is swollen. It is one type of otitis externa.

Fluoroquinolones are a relatively new class of antibiotics. Two examples of ear drops containing fluoroquinolones are CiproHC and Floxin Otic. These newer fluoroquinolone antibiotics are potent against any one bacteria and against many different bacteria.

Granulation tissue is fragile, fleshy, inflammatory tissue that can develop when an infection spreads beyond the ear canal and causes inflammatory tissue. It has a "raw" appearance. Often surgery is required if granulation tissue develops.

Hearing bones are the hammer (malleus), which is attached to the eardrum and to the anvil (incus). The anvil is attached to the stirrup (stapes).

Immature immunity describes individuals, especially young children and infants, who have lower resistance to infections than adults owing to the age difference between them.

Immunoglobulins are antibodies that fight off infections.

Infection indicates the presence of organisms, such as viruses or bacteria, that have caused an inflammation.

Inflammation is the body's response to injury or abnormal stimulation caused by viruses, bacteria, or physical or chemical agents.

Inner ear receives the sound from the eardrum and ossicles in the middle ear and also houses the balance mechanism (semicircular canals).

Isthmus is the narrow portion in the middle of the eustachian tube important in stopping nasopharyngeal secretions from getting into the middle ear.

Labyrinth is another term for the inner ear: both the cochlea (hearing) and the semicircular canals (balance) are housed here.

Labyrinthitis is an infection of the inner ear, which contains the body's balance system and hearing apparatus. Symptoms include dizziness, poor balance, and a moderate to severe hearing loss.

Lumen is the channel in the eustachian tube through which air passes into the middle ear, and secretions in the middle ear go into the nasopharynx.

Lymphadenopathy is enlarged glands. Lymphadenopathy is rare in swimmer's ear.

Mastoid is connected to and behind the middle ear and is composed of many air cells, which resemble Swiss cheese. You can feel the outer bony part of the mastoid on your head behind the outer ear.

Mastoidectomy is opening the mastoid behind the ear and draining infection.

Meningitis is an infection involving the membrane covering the brain.

Middle ear is the space behind the eardrum, between the outer ear and inner ear, and connected to the eustachian tube in front and the mastoid behind.

Middle ear air cushion is the normal backpressure of air in the middle ear that keeps unwanted secretions in the nasopharynx from getting into the middle ear through the eustachian tube.

Middle ear effusion is the liquid resulting from acute otitis media or otitis media with effusion. The effusion may be thin and watery, thick and mucus-like, or pus-like.

Myringotomy is a tiny hole made in the eardrum by a little knife or needle to remove and drain middle ear fluid.

Nasopharynx is the open area behind the nasal cavities, the back of the nose. It connects to the throat.

Oligosaccharides are sugar-like compounds that work by preventing bacteria from attaching to the nasopharynx, which, in turn, prevents the bacteria from spreading to the middle ear. They are currently being studied as a way to prevent otitis media.

Ossicles (hearing bones) are the three smallest bones in the body, which are connected to each other and transmit sound from the eardrum to the inner ear. They are the **malleus** (shaped like a hammer), **incus** (shaped like an anvil), and **stapes** (shaped like the stirrup of a riding saddle).

Otalgia is ear pain or earache and is the main symptom of swimmer's ear.

Otitis externa means, literally, "outer ear." It is sometimes called "swimmer's ear."

Otitis media means, literally, "inflammation of the middle ear."

Otitis media with effusion is an inflammation of the middle ear in which a collection of liquid is present in the middle ear space; there is no perforation of the eardrum. It is also called **serous otitis media**.

Otitis prone defines those individuals who are susceptible to getting ear infections.

Otolaryngologist is an ear, nose, and throat doctor.

Otorrhea is any liquid that drains out of the ear. During an ear infection, this liquid is usually a thick green or yellow pus.

Otoscopy is a procedure used to determine if fluid is in the middle ear. The doctor uses an **otoscope** to examine the eardrum and some parts of the middle ear.

Outer ear (pinna or **auricle)** is the cup-shaped structure on either side of the head (where earrings are put).

Patulous eustachian tube is an abnormally open (patent) eustachian tube.

Perforation is a hole (in the eardrum). Perforations can be **acute** (when an eardrum ruptures during an attack of acute otitis media or when a tympanostomy tube falls out of the eardrum and the eardrum does not heal) or **chronic** (when a perforation does not close by itself within 2 to 3 months after occurring).

pH level is the balance between acid and alkaline. The normal pH level of the outer ear is to be more acid than alkaline. The normal pH level of most swimming pools is to be more alkaline than acid, which is why swimming often causes swimmer's ear.

Rebound is chronic congestion of the nose owing to overuse of nose-drop decongestants.

Reflux is the abnormal backward flow of secretions up the eustachian tube into the middle ear.

Resistance (bacteria) means that bacteria have managed to change in such a way that some antibiotics cannot kill them. Not all bacteria are resistant, and when they are resistant, some antibiotics will still kill them.

Resistance (human) is the body's ability to fight off infection.

Retraction pocket is a dimple-like defect in the eardrum caused by one part of the eardrum being pulled (retracted) into the middle ear by persistent middle ear negative pressure owing to abnormal eustachian tube function.

Runny ear is like a "runny" nose; the liquid that comes from the ear looks like what comes out of the nose during a cold or sinusitis.

Semicircular canals are in the inner ear (labyrinth) and are involved in balance.

Sensorineural hearing loss is caused by damage to the inner ear hearing mechanism (the cochlea), hearing nerve, or hearing part of the brain.

Sequela (plural, **sequelae**) is a condition that follows an illness as a consequence of it.

Sinusitis is a potential cause of otitis media. Symptoms include face pain or headache, a runny nose, a daytime cough, foul breath, a cold lasting longer than 2 weeks, or, when fever is present, similar to a severe cold.

Skull base osteomyelitis is a very serious condition occurring when infection spreads from the outer ear to the base of the skull. It is one type of otitis externa. Usually some other underlying condition such as diabetes or acquired immune deficiency syndrome (AIDS) is present.

Swimmer's ear is a common name for otitis externa. However, *swimmer's ear* is really just one type of otitis externa. Its medical name is *acute bacterial otitis externa*.

Tinnitus is hearing abnormal sounds in the ear, such as ringing, buzzing, popping, and snapping.

Tonsillectomy is surgical removal of the tonsils.

Tonsils are the two ball-like lymphoid structures that are on either side of the throat.

Tympanocentesis is the procedure used to determine which type of bacteria is causing an infection in the middle ear. It is done by putting a needle, attached to a syringe, through the eardrum into the middle ear and suctioning out the fluid, which is then tested in the laboratory.

Tympanometry is a procedure used to determine if fluid is in the middle ear. It works by sending sound through a stopper that is put into the ear canal. The doctor uses a **tympanometer** to perform the procedure, and a **tympanogram** is a visual recording of the sound that bounces off the eardrum.

Tympanosclerosis is scarring of the eardrum caused by recurrent otitis media, a tympanostomy tube, or both.

Tympanostomy tube is a little plastic tube that is inserted into a tiny hole in the eardrum to aerate the middle ear.

Vaccines are usually given in a shot to prevent infection, such as the *Haemophilus influenzae* type b (HIB) vaccine.

Vertigo is a subjective sensation of movement of the patient or the surroundings.

HIV infection, as risk factor for otitis media, 21
Host-related risk factors, for otitis media, 18–23, 19t

Immunity
  immature, 157
  as risk factor for otitis media, 21–22
Immunoglobulins, 157
Incus, 159
Infection
  bacterial
    in chronic suppurative otitis media, 88–89, 90t
    in otitis externa, 121–122, 126
    in otitis media, 50, 51f, 52
  defined, 157
  fungal, in otitis externa, 122–123
  viral
    in otitis externa, 123
    in otitis media, 46–48, 48f, 50, 50f
    in upper respiratory infection, 23–24
Inflammation, 157
  corticosteroids for, 136–137
Inflation of the eustachian tube, 73
Inner ear, 157
Intracranial complications, of otitis media, 16t, 111–114, 112f
  brain abscess, 113–114
  extradural abscess, 112–113
  focal otitic encephalitis, 113
  meningitis, 111–112
  otitic hydrocephalus, 114
  sigmoid sinus thrombosis, 15, 114
  signs and symptoms of, 87t
  subdural abscess, 113
Intracranial hypertension, benign, 15, 114
Intratemporal (extracranial) complications, of otitis media, 15t–16t, 85–111
Intravenous therapy, antibiotic, 94–96
Isthmus, 157

Keratoma, defined, 13

Labyrinth, defined, 157
Labyrinthine sclerosis, 105
Labyrinthitis
  as complication of otitis media, 104–105
  defined, 13, 157

serous, 104–105
  suppurative, 105
Lateral sinus thrombosis, 15, 114
Lorabid, 63t
Loracarbef (Lorabid), 63t
Lumen, defined, 157
Lymphadenopathy, defined, 157

Macrolides, 63t
Malignant otitis externa, 119, 144
Malleus, 159
Mastoid, defined, 158
Mastoidectomy, defined, 158
Mastoiditis
  acute
    with cellulitis, 101, 103
    as complication of otitis media, 100–103
    defined, 153
    osteitis, 101, 102f, 103
    with periosteitis, 100–101
    without periosteitis/osteitis, 100
  chronic, 104
  as complication of otitis media, 100
  defined, 12
  masked, 103
  subacute, 103
Meningitis, 14, 111–112, 158
Middle ear, 158
Middle ear air cushion, 158
Middle ear effusion
  defined, 11, 158
  otitis media with. See Effusion, otitis media with
  persistent
    defined, 12
    management, 65–66
    signs and symptoms of, 54
Middle ear system, anatomy of, 33f
Minimum inhibitory concentration (MIC), 133
Moraxella catarrhalis, 154
  in otitis media, 50, 51f, 52, 55
  resistance issues with, 134
  vaccination for, 150
Motor disturbance, as complication of otitis media, 98
Myringitis, bullous, 123
Myringosclerosis, 77f, 110
Myringotomy, 57–58, 158. *See also* Tympanostomy tube placement
  in acute otitis media, 59–60
  indications for, 57t, 59